HALI TO SIS

A PUBLIC HEALTH PERSPECTIVE

HALITOSIS

A PUBLIC HEALTH PERSPECTIVE

Sonia Raina

First published by
Papertowns Publishers
72, Vishwanath Dham Colony,
Niwaru Road, Jhotwara,
Jaipur, 302012

Halitosis: A Public Health Perspective
Copyright © Sonia Raina, 2022

ISBN Print Book – 978-93-94670-03-7

Cover by Neha Agrawal
nehaa.2089@gmail.com

Content

Halitosis is a medical term first coined by the Listerine Company in 1921, used to describe unpleasant breath, regardless of its sources, oral or non-oral.[1] The word originates from the Latin "halitus" meaning "breath" and the Greek "osis" meaning "abnormal" or "diseased".[2] Other terms used are bad or foul breath, breath malodour, oral malodour, foetor exore, and foetor oris and should not be confused with the generally temporary oral odour caused by intake of certain foods, tobacco, or medications.[3]

Knowledge of this condition dates back to ancient cultures. The Talmud, a collection of ancient rabbinical writings dating back more than two millennia, states that bad breath is a major disability.[2] Halitosis may be a valuable diagnostic aid, in fact, Hippocrates is credited with having cited the nose as "a true diagnostic guide"[4] and suggested a rinse using herbs and wine be used to sweeten the unpleasant odors of the breath.[5] It was believed that in perfect health the breath is almost odorless, but its ready modification by slight changes in the state of health makes it a valuable diagnostic aid. Local and systemic etiologic factors were listed based on clinical observation rather than scientific experiment. Earlier researchers also believed halitosis to be caused either by purely local factors or, by absorption of foul odors of the digestive system by saliva as the expired air passed through the mouth. Halitosis was thought to be a composite of odors due to digestion, metabolism, fermentation, and intra oral putrefaction, and that saliva is an excretion which acquires and excretes all iaceous odors.[4] In 1934, osmoscope was developed for measuring the intensity of odors in drinking water samples. Later it was used for breath analysis by Brening RH, Sulser GF and Fosdick LS in 1939.[4] Islam stresses the importance of fresh breath as part of good oral hygiene. Ladanum (mastic) are derived from the 'Pistacia lentiscus' tree used in the Mediterranean region for breath freshening for thousands of years, has been mentioned in the book of Genesis. Parsley, cloves, guava peels and egg shells have been considered as traditional remedies for bad breath in various countries across the world.[6]

During the last 40 years, our scientific knowledge about the source and causes of halitosis has become much greater. In 2002, Time magazine hailed Listerine's PocketPaks — the first breath strips that dissolved on the tongue — as one of their "Products of the Year" along with breakthroughs such as the birth control patch. Almost $1billion a year is spent in the United States on deodorant type mouth rinses, mints, and related over the counter products to manage bad breath.[7]

The overall prevalence of oral malodor in the adult population is uncertain. Bad breath is a common condition found in approximately 50% of the adult population as a severe chronic problem.[6] Most individuals experience personal discomfort and social embarrassment leading to emotional distress. The consequences of oral malodor may be more than social; it may signal the presence of disease. In recent years the aetiology of halitosis has become increasingly clear, and it is now known that halitosis originates more from within the oral cavity than elsewhere in the body. Halitosis is not a disease but rather a symptom of underlying oral, systemic or psychological conditions. The primary cause of halitosis is due to the release of odoriferous volatile sulphur compounds (VSC) in the exhaled air. Therefore, more than any other health professional, dentists ought to be well informed on halitosis in order to provide effective treatment and proper advice to the significant proportion of the general population affected by this condition.[5] Although more than 200 volatile compounds are found in human breath, only volatile sulfur compounds have been found to have a good correlation between concentration and organoleptic values.[8]

The three primary measurement method of halitosis are organoleptic measurement, gas chromatography, sulphide monitoring. The scientific and practical value of additional or alternative measurement methods, such as BANA test, chemical sensors, salivary incubation test, has to be established.[3]

Before treating oral malodor the dental practitioner should assess all oral diseases and conditions that may contribute to oral malodor. Methods that have proven their effectiveness to a variable level are tongue cleaning, specifically the dorso-posterior region of the tongue, mechanical reduction of micro-organisms through improved oral hygiene procedures, toothpastes containing triclosan and a copolymer or sodium bicarbonate. A successful in-vitro test of lethal photosensitization of two common oral pathogens with high intensity red filtered halogen 1 amphasal so been achieved and can prove to be a valuable treatment modality.[9] Periodontal treatment is required because periodontal conditions contribute to oral pathological halitosis and although dental caries may not be a significant cause of oral malodour, caries treatment is recommended.[1] Recent research on oral malodor has revived the dental professions interest in this area and the increase in research and interest in oral malodor among dental professionals should result in a better understanding of the etiology of oral malodor and the development of more effective diagnostic and treatment methods.[10]

EPIDEMIOLOGY

There are rather few community based studies which have attempted to document the prevalence of oral malodor. Furthermore, those studies that exist have used differing methodologies and outcome measures such as self-reported oral malodor, or objective measurement, for example, by measurement of volatile sulphur compounds.[11] A nearly study from The Netherlands among 11,625 individuals revealed a prevalence of approximately 25% in subjects older than 60 years. In subjects under 20 years, the prevalence of oral halitosis was 10%, indicating that the prevalence of this condition increases with age.[2] In a Swedish study of 840 men, oral malodor as assessed by clinical assessment was only present in around 2% of the population.[11] In contrast, a large Japanese study of more than 2600 subjects assessed by Volatile Sulfur Compound monitor found the prevalence of malodor above 20%. Similarly, a study of 2500 subjects in China reported an overall prevalence of malodor of 27.5%, which was particularly associated with the presence of tongue coating.[11]

A recent Brazilian study of the prevalence of oral malodor assessed its presence by surveying University students (as "informants") regarding the prevalence of persisting malodor in members of their households. This was an interesting methodology as it overcomes the limitations of self-reporting of malodor whilst retaining the subjective judgment of malodor; the design might also facilitate the recruitment of large numbers of subjects. In this study approximately 15% of the population of a total of 344 subjects had informant-reported oral malodor. In all these studies no association was found between increased age and oral malodor.[11] According to national Survey 1999 in Japan the prevalence of individuals with complaint of halitosis is approximately 14% and in United States, it is estimated that 10-30% of the adult population have and appreciable problem with bad breath.[2]

There is a relative paucity of good clinical data describing the epidemiology of the condition, its social consequences, and lack of systematic guidelines for patient management. Studies in these are complicated by a number of factors which may complicate study design and the collection of reliable clinical data. Firstly, clinically significant oral malodor is ultimately a subjective response to the presence of unpleasant or volatile substances in the breath. This may complicate diagnostic criteria and outcome measures in intervention studies. Secondly, oral malodor is difficult for an individual to assess themselves, and indeed a significant number of cases of self-reported oral malodor cannot be verified by objective measures. Thirdly, the condition may be a source of personal embarrassment and thus recruitment of affected individuals may be difficult. This also leads to the possibility of ascertainment bias in clinical studies where recruitment may typically come from self-referred subjects to dedicated multidisciplinary oral malodor clinics.[11]

Overall, the epidemiological data support the view that in many populations oral malodor may be present in greater than 10% of the population, and possibly markedly higher than this. More precise figures may require many further large investigations, but are unlikely to be directly generalisable to other communities.[11]

There are two widely used indices for the organoleptic assessment of halitosis. One described by Rosenberg et al.[12] and second by Seemann[13] Index described by Rosenberg et al.[12]

Grade 0 = no appreciable odor.

Grade 1 = barely noticeable odor.

Grade 2 = slight but clearly noticeable odor.

Grade 3 = moderate odor.

Grade 4 = strong odor.

Grade 5 = extremely foul odor.

Index described by Seemann[13]

Grade 0: halitosis not detected.

Grade 1: halitosis only diagnosed when the subject was breathing through an open mouth and the observer approached to a distance of about 10 cm.

Grade 2: Halitosis only detected at a distance of about 30 cm from the subject's mouth.

Grade 3: Halitosis already diagnosed on welcoming the subject, with a distance of approximately 1 m between the examiner's nose and the subject's mouth.

PHYSIOLOGY

The expired air of non-halitosis patients contains upto 150 different molecules. The perception of these molecules depends on the following factors:

a. The odor itself (*olfactory response*) can be pleasant, unpleasant, or even repulsive.

b. Each particular molecule has its specific concentration before it can be detected

(*threshold concentration*)

c. The *odor power* is the extent of concentration that must be increased before a malodor judge will give it a higher odor score.

d. The *volatility* of the compound is the concentration at which it escapes from the liquid phase into the air.

The odor power is strongest for hydrogen sulfide, methyl mercaptan and dimethyl sulfide; that is, if the concentration of these products increases five fold to ten fold, the odor will receive a higher organoleptic rating. For the other compounds, increases of 25 to 100 times are needed to reach a similar effect. Skatole and methyl mercaptan are detected at the lowest concentration. The three sulfide products have the lowest volatility (i.e., will escape the liquid phase first).

(Table I)[7]

Table I: Odor Threshold and Odor Power of Key Malodorous Compounds

Compound	Odor thresholds		Odor power	Volatility (Henry's Constants)
	Greenman $(mol.dm^{-3})$	*Devos* $(mol.dm^{-3})$	*Greenman(x increase to "up"score 1 unit)*	*Volatility (Kcc)inH$_2$O at20^{0}C*
Butyrate	2.3×10^{-10}	2.4×10^{-10}	10-fold	3.9×10^4
Isovalerate	1.8×10^{-11}	2.5×10^{-11}	42-fold	2.5×10^4
Skatole	7.2×10^{-11}	1.0×10^{-12}	8-fold	4.1×10^5
Trimethylamine	1.8×10^{-11}	1.5×10^{-11}	96-fold(low affinity)	2.0×10^2
Putrescine	9.1×10^{-10}	1.0×10^{-9}	27-fold	4.1×10^1
Dimethylsulfide	5.9×10^{-8}	5.0×10^{-8}	10-fold	1.7×10^1
Hydrogensulfide	6.4×10^{-10}	5.0×10^{-10}	4.8fold	$\sim 1.7 \times 10^1$
Methylmercaptan	1.0×10^{-11}	1.0×10^{-11}	7.2fold	$\sim 1.7 \times 10^1$

ETIOPATHOGENESIS

Assessing causation is a dubious duty. Causes of bad breath can be multiple, and etiological culprits may shift overtime. Ninety percent of the time, the dark, wet and warm oral cavity is the source of malodor (localized); systemic origin comprises roughly the remaining ten percent of cases. It has been reported that sulfur-containing volatiles are the central elements of oral malodor and that their levels correlate with oral malodor intensity determined organoleptically.[19] These Volatile Sulfur Compounds are the predominant elements of oral malodor, but other odorous volatiles, such as certain amines and fatty acids, may also play a role.[20] Most frequent sources of halitosis (80–90%) exist within the oral cavity and include bacterial reservoirs such as the dorsum of the tongue, saliva and periodontal pockets, where anaerobic bacteria degrade sulphur-containing amino acids to produce the foul smelling Volatile Sulfur Compounds.[20] Three factors are involved in the aetiology of halitosis, namely the bacteria that produce the malodorous compounds, the substrates that the bacteria utilize to release the odor compounds, and the malodorous compounds themselves. In the absence of anyone of these factors halitosis is unlikely to occur.[6]

BACTERIA

The oral cavity is an ideal location for many microorganisms to flourish. It has various sheltered areas such as interdental spaces, dental caries, gingival sulcus and deeper layers of papillae on the dorsum of the tongue, which function as bacterial reservoirs. Microorganisms thrive not only in these sheltered areas but also on all the surfaces in the oral cavity, including the non-shedding surfaces such as on teeth and restorations. They are also present in saliva and in the gingival crevicular fluid (GCF)[6] but the non-shedding surfaces of the teeth offer a far different habitat than the continually shedding surfaces of the oral musosa.[21]

Several investigators have identified the Gram-negative bacterial component of the oral micro flora as mainly responsible for oral malodor production.[19] This relationship was demonstrated convincingly by McNamara et al.[22] when they found that

(1) the rise in odor in whole saliva incubated with no added sugar is matched by a rise in the ratio of Gram-negative to Gram-positive organisms;

(2) if glucose is added at a concentration of 20

millimolar to make the pH acidic, the suppressed odor formation that results is matched by emergence of a flora composed predominantly of Gram- positive organisms; and

(3) if glucose is added at only 2 millimolar, a concentration too low to prevent the saliva from becoming alkaline, odor formation once more occurs and is accompanied by a microbial shift in favor of the Gram-negative members of the oral flora. The Gram-positive bacteria in the mouth depend largely upon carbohydrates as their main energy source for growth, which they can get readily from fermentable carbohydrates provided in the diet. In contrast, the Gram- negative bacterial population derives energy from both carbohydrates and protein sources. Thus it is to be expected that Gram-negative bacteria would be selected and odor formation produced when no or only insufficient glucose or other fermentable carbohydrates are added to incubated saliva, and with carbohydrate addition Gram positive bacteria would be selected.

Organisms responsible for the hydrolysis of peptides and proteins, and the production of volatile sulphur-containing compounds include proteolytic obligate anaerobes, especially the Gram-negative species, mainly retained in tongue coating and periodontal pockets.[3] At present, it has been estimated that approximately 700 species, including phylotypes, could inhabit the human oral cavity[21] with atleast 150 different species being present at anytime.[5] Bacteria known to produce volatile sulphur- containing compounds include *Aggregati bacteractinomycetemcomitans* (formerly *Actinobacillus actinomycetemcomitans*), *Actinomyces* species, *Atopobium parvulum, Campylobacter rectus, Desulfovibrio* species, *Eikenella corrodens, Eubacterium sulci, Fusobacterium species, Peptostreptococcus micros, Porphyromonas endodontalis, Porphyromonas gingivalis, Prevotella*species, *Solobacterium moorei, Tannerellaforsythia* (formerly *Bacteriodesforsythus* or *Tannerellaforsythensis*), *Treponemadenticola, Veillonella*species, *Vibrio* species, a phylotype of *Dialister*, a phylotype of the uncultivated phylum, and a phylotype of *Streptococcus*, and as yet unidentified sulphur-reducing bacteria. The species diversity found in halitosis samples suggests that halitosis may be the result of complex interactions between several bacterial species.[3]

Helicobacter pylori has been suggested as a cause of halitosis, and can produce volatile sulfur compounds. Although some have not found an association between functional dyspepsia, peptic ulcer disease and *Helicobacter pylori* infection with halitosis occurrence or severity.[23]

Many theories have been put forward by which microbial etiology of halitosis can be explained. Kleinberg I et al.[24] suggested that there are three areas of evidence to consider the bacteria present in the oral cavity as the most likely origin of halitosis. First, in vitro, oral organic substrates and bacteria produced the odorous compounds. In vivo, production of volatile sulphur-containing compounds was induced upon provision of peptides and amino acids in the mouth. Second, halitosis was immediately reduced by reduction of substrates and micro-organisms, such as brushing the teeth and cleaning the tongue, which would not have been possible if the halitosis originated in non-oral regions, such as the nose, the tonsils, the lungs, or the stomach. Third, antibacterial agents reduce halitosis. According to Scully Cand Greenman J[23] two theories of microbial etiology can be proposed: a specific theory (that just a few single species are etiological and capable of causing malodor; their presence solely will explain malodor) and a nonspecific theory, which suggests that many species (most being strict anaerobes) have the ability to biotransform substrates into volatile compounds or volatile sulfur compounds and that many groups can therefore substitute for others; there is no single causative species. The tongue has the largest bacterial load of any oral tissue and makes the greatest contribution to bacteria found in saliva.[2]

THE SUBSTRATES

An organic substance that is acted upon in a biochemical reaction is called a substrate. The consumed food is acted upon in a similar manner by various digestive enzymes and in a way becomes the substrate. Bacteria resident in the oral cavity utilize part of the food that is stagnant in the mouth as their substrate. However, only water-soluble nutrients enter the bacteria through pores on the cell wall, and are then digested within the cell. In contrast, complex molecules, such as proteins or complex carbohydrates, are broken down into simple molecules outside the bacteria by enzymes before they are transported across the cell membrane. Following the proteolytic activity of bacteria on the sulphur-containing amino acid substrates such as cystine, cysteine and methionine, the end products released are the odoriferous Volatile Sulfur Compounds that are associated with halitosis. However, if a mainly carbohydrate nutrient is present, bacterial putrefaction lowers the pH to an acid medium and Volatile Sulfur Compounds formation is inhibited.

The substrates for this putrefaction process come from stagnant food, exfoliated epithelial cells, effused leukocytes, stagnant saliva, gingival crevicular fluid and inflammatory exudates.[5]

MALODOR COMPOUNDS

The human breath has been found to contain more than 200 volatile compounds, including Volatile Sulfur Compounds, gases not containing sulphur such as amines (cadaverine), volatile aromatic compounds (indole, skatole) and short chain carboxylic acids (SCCA), andorganic acids (acetic, proprionic). However, contrary to the traditional belief that ammonia and amines were the main source of halitosis, it was Tonzetichand Richter[25] who first reported that Volatile Sulfur Compounds are the main components of halitosis. Of the total Volatile Sulfur Compounds found in the mouth air, 90% is made up of hydrogen sulphide, methyl mercaptan and to a lesser extent dimethyl sulphide. However, the Volatile Sulfur Compounds that cause the halitosis of oral origin differ from Volatile Sulfur Compounds found in blood borne halitosis of extra oral origin. Compounds such as methyl mercaptan and hydrogen sulphide that are associated with oral malodour are not found in blood-borne halitosis. The breath of a person with halitosis of extraoral origin may rarely contain odoriferous amines.

Table II lists some of the common odour-producing compounds along with their odour recognition threshold concentration. The malodour gases with the lowest recognition threshold concentration such as allyl mercaptan are the most odorous, whereas odour compounds such as ammonia have the least odour.[5]

Table II: Breath Malodour Compounds and Their Characteristics

Name	Formula	Odour Characteristics	100% Odour recognition
Allyl mercaptan	CH2=CHCH2SH	garlic-like pungent,	0.05ppb*
Propylmercaptan	CH3CH2CH2SH	unpleasant pungent	0.70ppb
Dimethyldisulphide	CH3SSCH3	pungent, rotten cabbage	7.00ppb
Methylmercaptan	CH3SH	unpleasantly sweet	35.00ppb
DimethylSulfide	CH3SCH3	slightly pungent rotten	100.00ppb
Carbondisulphide	CS3	eggs	1000.00ppb
HydrogenSulfide	H2S (CH3)3N	fishy, ammoniacal	4000.00ppb
Trimethylamine	(CH3)2NH	fishy, ammonical	6000.00ppb
Dimethylamine	NH3	pleasantly sweet	55,000.00ppb

ppb, parts per billion

Gram-negative, proteolytic bacteria are believed to play an essential role in the formation of Volatile Sulfur Compounds, although Gram-positive bacteria such as Peptostreptococcus species have also shown ability to produce Volatile Sulfur Compounds in vitro.[2] These anaerobes produce malodor volatile compounds in many instances, **(Table III)** which include the following:[23]

- Volatile sulfur compounds, mainly methyl mercaptan and hydrogen sulfide, which are the main contributors to intra-oral halitosis. The volatile sulfur compound, dimethyl sulfide, is the main contributor to extra-oral or blood-borne halitosis but may also contribute to oral malodor.
- Short-chain fatty acids (butyric, valeric and propionic acids).
- Polyamines (putrescine and cadaverine).
- Acetone, 2-butanone, 2-pentanone and 1-propanol are common to all volunteers with halitosis and are present in both alveolar (lung) and mouth air; indole and dimethyl selenide are present in alveolar air.

Table III: Odoriferous Components That Can Give Rise to Oral Malodor

Volatile sulfur compounds	• Methyl mercaptan • Hydrogen sulfide • Dimethyl sulfide
Diamines	• Putrescine • Cadaverine
Short-chain fattyacids	• Butyric acid • Valeric acid • Propionic acid
Indoles	• Indole • Methyl-indole (skatole)

Tonzetich and Richter[25] divided the volatiles produced into three fractions: acidic, basic, and neutral. The acidic fraction contained odorous volatiles that collectively gave the incubating saliva its putrid odor. These volatiles were mainly sulfur-containing compounds and included hydrogen sulfide, methyl mercaptan, and, to a much lesser extent, dimethyl sulfide. Ammonia, one of the major end products of amino acid degradation by the oral bacteria, was found in the basic volatile fraction. It was not odorous. When several sulfur-containing substrates, which included cysteine, cystine, methionine, reduced and oxidized glutathione, and peptones, were incubated with whole saliva, odor intensity increased considerably. Cystine and oxidized glutathione showed delays, which is consistent with disulfide to thiol conversion being an essential first step before these sulfur-containing substrates can produce malodorous volatiles **(Fig I)**. This conversion is favored by Nicotinamide adenine dinucleotide (NADH) and Nicotinamide adenine dinucleotide dehydrogenase and reduced conditions that favor formation of the Nicotinamide adenine dinucleotide needed by cystine and oxidized glutathione to produce cysteine and reduced glutathione, respectively. Cysteine degradation catalyzed by cysteine desulfhydrase will yield Hydrogen Sulfide, ammonia, and pyruvate. Methionine, after deamination, can result in the formation of methyl mercaptan and α-ketobutyrate. In the presence of serine, methionine may also yield cysteine and, in turn, hydrogen sulfide. According to various studies conducted, it appears that methyl mercaptan is the predominant causative factor of malodor.[2] Despite the strong evidence that volatile sulfur compounds are the major causative factors in intraoral halitosis, several research groups still suggest that other volatile compounds such as cadaverine (produced from the decarboxylation of lysine), indole, skatole, and butyric acid may influence oral halitosis.[2] Cadaverine and putrescineare common bacterial degradation products. Cadaverine previously shown to be a component of human dental plaque is a malodorous product of bacterial putrefaction of meat and fish and may be produced in saliva as the result of decarboxylation (i.e, of lysine and ornithine) or, in the case of putrescine, by transamination.[26] Tonzetich[27] showed that diamines, such as cadaverine, inhibited odor formation. He also stated that indole and skatole, although emanating an objectionable odor in pure state, did not impart an odor to saliva under conditions approximating those of the oral cavity and ascribed this to their extremely low volatility. The same holds for butyric acid. Due to their low volatilities these compounds have a low odor potential. This is in strong contrast with the volatile sulfur compounds which have a very high odor potential.[2] Saliva may also be a source of oral malodor especially as a result of the degradation of amino acids by Gram- negative microorganisms. Salivary proteins contain sulphate, but few sulfur containing aminoacids. Nevertheless, volatile sulfur compounds are still produced from salivary proteins.[28] The volatile sulfur compound, dimethyl sulfide is the main contributor toextra-oral orblood-borne halitosis Dimethyl sulfide mayalsocome from methionine. Dimethyl sulphide, which is a neutral compound that is also stable in blood, can be blood-borne and release dint othe lung air. Thus in patients with a cirrhotic liver the odour named fetor hepaticus is caused by dimethyl sulphide.[5]

FIGURE I: Metabolic Pathways Involved In Methionine, Cysteine, and Cystine Degradation During Odor Formation

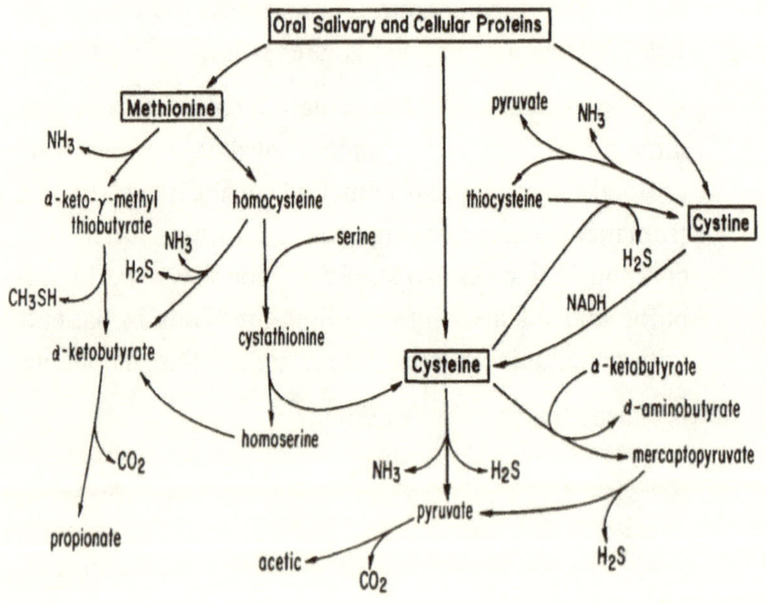

In contrast to Hydrogen Sulfide which is present in the greatest concentration in mouth air, measurements of Volatile Sulfur Compounds within periodontal pockets have demonstrated that methyl mercaptan is often the predominant compound. It has been reported that the ratios of methyl mercaptan to hydrogen sulfide are moderately increased in deeper pockets.[29] However, increases in these ratios were greatest and most highly correlated with disease when pockets were segregated using presence or absence of bleeding on probing. These data would indicate that the presence of methyl mercaptan within a periodontal pocket may be associated with active periodontal disease.

Tongue coatings when incubated with casein, the levels of certain compounds increased and new ones appeared, including nine additional sulfur-containing compounds. As thorough as this analysis was, it did not detect the diamines, cadaverine or putrescine, or most of them alodorous fatty acids, such as isobutyric, propionic, isopropionic, and valeric acids that are produced by the anaerobic flora characteristic of the tongue and periodontal pockets. The detection of new compounds arising after the addition of case into the tongue coatings raises the possibility that the production of malodorous compounds is dynamic, changing in response to the nutrient source.[30] This phenomenon has also been studied invitro using a salivary sediment system in which saliva is centrifuged and then suspended in a small volume.[30] But what was most interesting was the observation that the production of malodorous molecules was inhibited by an acid environment, which occurred when glucose was added to the mixture. This observation, which has implications for the control of malodor, can be explained by therapidity by which glucose is fermented by the saccharolytic flora such as the streptococci and actinomyces, which are the numerically dominant organisms in saliva, to form the acidic pH values that would inhibit the metabolic activity of many proteolytic species. Also, the phenomenon of glucose catabolite repression would cause such species as *Fusobacteria nucleatum* and *Prevotella intermedia*, which can ferment both carbohydrates and peptides, to preferentially use carbohydrates, if both substrates are available.

CLASSIFICATION OF HALITOSIS

I. Based on etiological factors (Dominic et al.)[31]

1. Local factors of pathologic origin
2. Local factors of non-pathologic origin
3. Systemic factors of pathologic origin
4. Systemic factors of non-pathologic origin
5. Halitosis due to systemic administration of drugs
6. Halitosis due to xerostomia

II. Based on Source of Origin (Dayan et al.)[32]

1. Odor emanating within oral cavity
2. Odor emanating from regions immediately adjacent oral cavity
3. Odor emanating from lungs

III. Based on sites of origin (Bogdasarian)[33]

1. Normal breath and physiologic mouth odor
2. Odors from oral conditions
3. Odors from nasopharynx, pharynx, lungs
4. Odor secreted from the lungs.

IV. Based on Types (Miyazaki et al.)[34]

I. Genuine halitosis

a. Physiologic Halitosis b. Pathologic Halitosis
(i) Oral
(ii) Extraoral
II. Pseudohalitosis
III. Halitophobia

I. Genuine Halitosis- Obvious malodour, with intensity beyond socially acceptable level, is perceived.

a. Physiologic Halitosis- Malodor arises through putrefactive process within the oral cavity. Neither specific disease nor pathologic condition that could cause halitosis is found. Origin is mainly the dorso posterior region of the tongue. Temporary halitosis due to dietary factors (e.g.,garlic) is excluded.

b. Pathologic Halitosis.
1. Oral- Halitosis caused by disease, pathologic condition or malfunction of oral tissues.

Main oral causes of halitosis are:[23]

i. Plaque-related gingival and periodontal disease- Gingivitis, periodontitis, acute necrotizing ulcerative gingivitis, pericoronitis, abscesses

ii. Ulceration- Systemic disease (inflammatory /
infectious disorders, cutaneous, gastrointestinal
and hematological disease), malignancy, local
causes, aphthae, drugs

iii. Hyposalivation- e.g. from drugs, Sjögren's
syndrome, radiotherapy, chemotherapy

iv. Tongue coating- Poor hygiene

v. Wearing dental appliances- Poor hygiene

vi. Dental conditions- Food packing

vii. Bone diseases- Jaw dry sockets, osteomyelitis,
osteonecrosis, malignancy

2. *Extraoral*- conditions and diseases that do not
affect primarily the oral cavity Main extra-oral
causes of halitosis are:[23]

(i) Respiratory system– Sinusitis, Antral
malignancy, Cleft palate, Foreign bodies in the
nose, Nasal malignancy, Tonsilloliths,
Tonsillitis, Pharyngeal malignancy, Lung
infections, Bronchitis, Bronchiectasis, Lung
malignancy.

(i) Gastrointestinal Tract- Esophageal
diverticulum, Gastro-esophageal reflux
disease, Malignancy.

(ii) Metabolic disorders- Acetone-like smell in
uncontrolled diabetes, Uremic breath in renal
failure, Foetorhepaticusin liver disease,

Trimethylaminuria, Hypermethioninemia, Cystinosis.

(iii) Drugs- amphetamines, chloralhydrate, cytotoxic agents, dimethyl sulphoxide, disulfiram, nitrates and nitrites, phenothiazines, solvent abuse

II. Pseudo-halitosis- Obvious malodor is not perceived by others, although the patient stubbornly complains of its existence. Condition is improved by counselling (using literature support, education and explanation of examination results) and simple oral hygiene measures.

III. Halitophobia - After treatment for genuine halitosis or pseudo-halitosis, the patient persists in believing that he/she has halitosis. No physical or social evidence exists to suggest that halitosis is present.

ORAL CAUSES OF HALITOSIS

(A) Plaque-related gingival and periodontal disease

Gingivitis and Periodontitis

Plaque is composed of cells, mostly bacterial, within a matrix believed to be composed mostly of salivary protein and bacterial large-molecular-weight products. The loose outer most layer of the plaque in situ, often referred to as material alba, usually contains desquamated epithelial cells and blood cell elements. These cells and their debris are good sources of sulfur-containing substrates for odor production. The innermost region of the plaque may have an acquired pellicle, but this is probably low in sulfur-containing amino acids, since it originates mostly from salivary glycoprotein and bacterial cell walls. Gram-negative bacteria in plaque, the microbial component best able to putrefy the substrates that produce odorous volatiles, depend upon its state of maturation. Arise in Gram-negative bacteria usually occurs as plaque thickens; this coincides with the rise in the severity of gingivitis/periodontitis.[19] the low oxygen tension in deep periodontal pockets also results in a low pH and an activation of the decarboxylation of the amino acids (e.g., lysine, ornithine) to cadaverine and putrescine, two malodorous diamines.[35]

Acute Necrotizing Ulcerative Gingivitis

A characteristic and pronounced fetor exore is often associated with the disease, but can vary in intensity and in some cases is not very noticeable.[36]

Pericoronitis

The term pericoronitis refers to inflammation of the gingival in relation to the crown of an incompletely erupted tooth. It occurs most often in the mandibular third molar area. The symptoms of pericoronitis include a bad taste in the mouth (this often happens when there is an infection) and bad breath (halitosis) among others.[37]

Hyposalivation

Hyposalivation is associated with number of systemic diseases (Sjögren's syndrome, Rheumatoid arthritis) and is found to be higher among females and associated with the use of medications, such as antianginal, diuretics, antidepressants, and antiasthma, as well as thyroxine and is also a major complication of radiation or chemotherapy. Aging per se has no significant impact on salivary gland secretion. In the elderly, several factors, such as decrease of ptyalin, increase of mucin, and low stimulation of the peripheral receptors, have been implicated.[38] In the oral cavity, the thickness of the film or layer of saliva covering the oral surfaces after each swallow varies and appears to be least thick on the hard palate. The palate is the intra oral site where dryness is usually sensed first which facilitates volatilization of any odorous compounds generated by the bacteria and epithelial tissue on the palate. This should enable entry of these volatiles into the breath, especially during speech when air from the lungs streams over the palate. Thus, oral dryness might enable normally less volatile microbial end products to escape into the mouth air and contribute to the primary malodor produced by hydrogen sulfide and methyl mercaptan.[19]

Tongue coating

Research suggests that the tongue plays an important role in the production of oral malodor. The microbiota of the tongue surface is one of the most complex niches in human ecology, and approximately one-third of the bacterial population in the oral cavity is found on the tongue and not on other oral sites.[21] The dorsal tongue mucosa, shows a very irregular surface topography. The posterior part exhibits a number of oval cryptolymphatic units, which roughen the surface of this area. The anterior part is even rougher because of the high number of papillae present. These innumerable depressions in the tongue surfaces are ideal niches for bacterial adhesion and growth, sheltered from cleansing actions.[7] The filiform, circumvallate and foliate papillae and crevices associated with mucous glands and lingual tonsils increase the accumulation of bacteria and exfoliated epithelial cells by entrapping debris and retaining substrate, both of which favor the growth of anaerobic bacteria.[10] A fissured tongue (deep fissures on the dorsum, also called scrotal tongue or linguaplicata) and a hairy tongue (lingua villosa) have even a rougher surface. The accumulation of food remnants intermingled with exfoliated cells and bacteria causes a coating on the tongue dorsum. The latter cannot be easily removed because of the retention offered by their regular surface of the tongue dorsum. As such, the two factors essential for putrefaction are united.[30] The large surface area of the tongue exposed to the expired air, and the availability of substrates (nutrients) that can be degraded to malodorous molecules by the tongue flora make the tongue primary source to oral malodor relative to periodontal pockets found in periodontal disease. The large surface area of the tongue means that it can harbor high numbers of bacteria and this number would increase significantly when there is a coating.[30] The dorsum of tongue has therefore been considered as a primary source of oral malodor. Indeed, high correlations have been reported between tongue coating and odor formation.[7]

The tongue flora is exposed to the nutrients in about a litre of saliva per day compared to the 1 milliliter of gingival crevicular fluid that would bathe the periodontal plaque per day. The saliva would contain nutrients derived from the salivary glands, epithelial cells, gingival crevicular fluid, other bacteria, and food, accessed both during eating and later, if any food retained about the teeth is subsequently broken down. The tongue bacteria would have access to those nutrients present when blood from periodontal bleeding is admixed with saliva. Nutrients can be obtained directly from the mucosal surfaces, which are often ulcerated underneath the tongue coatings, thereby providing the odor-producing tongue bacteria with ready access to serum products. This access is likely to increase when the tongue is fissured, as the levels of components derived from the plasma and inflammatory cells are increased in saliva obtained from individuals with fissured tongues compared with saliva obtained from individuals without fissured tongues. Any inflammatory response in the tongue is likely to elicit increased production of endogenous beta defensins, which are cysteine-rich peptide antibiotics. If these peptides are degraded by the tongue flora, they would contribute to the volatile sulfur compounds found in patients with oral malodor.[30]

Despite the fact that the tongue has the largest bacterial load of any oral tissue and makes the greatest contribution to the bacteria found in the saliva, very little is known about the flora indigenous to the tongue. The tongue is colonized immediately after birth and anaerobic species, such as *Prevotella melaninogenicus* and *Fusobacterium nucleatum*, can be detected prior to the eruption of teeth. Their numbers and the presence of other anaerobes such as *Treponema denticola* and *Selenomonas* species increase at the time of the primary eruption of teeth. Young children (average age 4.2 years) with oral malodor had a significant increase in the salivary levels of *Prevotella oralis* and *Prevotella melaninogenica* compared with age-matched children without malodor, suggesting that this anaerobe was contributing to the malodor.[30] Presently new microorganisms are being discovered by direct amplification of microbial nucleic acids, and these techniques have doubled the number of bacterial species estimated to infect the human oral cavity.[39]

Different investigations have shown that the soft tissue surface can harbor periodontal pathogens.

Microbiota of the tongue has been characterized using culture and phase-contrast microscopy. The results showed that spirochetes, motile organisms, and black pigmented species, such as *Prevotella intermedia*, colonized the tongue. It was thus suggested that the presence of these organisms on the tongue surface could serve as an important ecological habitat for periodontal pathogens.[21] In addition, tongue of periodontally diseased and non-diseased young adult Kenyan subjects was examined.[21] The periodontal pathogens were present in both groups, although *Porphyromonas gingivalis* was detected significantly more frequently in tongue samples from periodontally diseased subjects. Microflora present on the tongue dorsum of subjects with and without halitosis was observed and it was found that the predominant species in test and control groups were *Veillonella sp.* and *Prevotella sp.* Greater species diversity was found in the halitosis samples compared with controls.[40]

The halitosis samples contained an increased incidence of unidentifiable Gram-negative rods, Gram-positive rods and Gram-negative coccobacilli. Perhaps the definite evidence that the tongue is the primary source of oral malodor came from studies in which volunteers were given mouth rinses containing cysteine, methionine or glutathione. Almost immediately a burst of volatile sulfur compounds in the exhaled air could be detected, with the largest amount coming from cysteine and the least from methionine. When aliquots of cysteine were placed for 30 seconds in discrete parts of the mouth, the greatest production of volatile sulfur compounds, from 1233 to 2500 ppb, came from the dorsum of the tongue, and lesser amounts from the buccal sulcus and sublingual areas. These studies were performed in individuals without malodor, so that even higher levels of volatile sulfur compounds would be expected to be produced in individuals with tongue coatings and fissured tongues. And this possibility was tested by giving subjects with and without oral malodor a 5% solution of trypticase, an enzymatic digest of casein (milk protein). Trypticase was chosen, as it was suspected that peptides derived from serum and the diet would be likely substrates for the proteolytic flora on the tongue. In subjects with malodor, the volatile sulfur compounds detected with the Halimeter increased from 367 ppb to 645 ppb within 120 seconds after the mouthrinse was expectorated. The corresponding value for subjects without malodor was an increase from 120 ppb to 174 ppb. This result clearly showed that subjects with malodor have a tongue flora that is readily capable of degrading sulfur containing peptides to malodorous volatile sulfur compounds.[30] Haraszthy VI et al.[39] conducted a study to identify the tongue bacteria using both anaerobic culture and direct amplification of 16 S ribosomal DNA and identified 4,088 isolates and phylotypes from the 13subjects, 32 species including 13 non cultivable species were found only in subjects with halitosis. **(Table IV).**[34]

TABLE IV: Most Prevalent Bacterial Species On The Human Tongue

BACTERIAL SPECIES	Prevalence (%)
Streptococcus salivarius	100
Prevotella melaninogenica	100
Streptococcus parasanguinis	100
Campylobacter concisus	88
Streptococcusmitis	100
Actinomyces odontolyticus	100
Prevotella species	63
Actinomyces Meyeri	88
Streptococcus oralis	100
Streptococcus infantis	63
Veillonella atypica	88
Streptococcus species	88
Veillonella dispar	88
Granulicatella adiacens	100
Streptococcus sanguinis	100
Fusobacterium nucleatum	75
Prevotella veroralis	75
Veillonella parvula	88
Rhodococcus opacus	25
Prevotella pallens	75
Gemella species oral strains	63

Dental Appliances

Acrylic dentures, especially when kept in the mouth at night or not regularly cleaned, can also produce a typical smell associated with candidiasis. The denture surface facing the gingival is porous and retentive for bacteria, yeasts, debris, and all factors that cause putrefaction.[7]

Dental Conditions

Possible causes within the dentition are deep carious lesions with food impaction and putrefaction, and a purulent discharge leading to important putrefaction. Interdental food impaction in large interdental areas and crowding of teeth favor food entrapment and accumulation of debris.[7]

Bone diseases

Dry Socket (alveolar osteitis) is a complication of wound healing following extraction of a tooth. Dry socket is characterized by detritus, grayish slough, severe pain and foul odor. The foul odor, in particular, is a result of the disintegration of the blood clot by putrefaction rather than by orderly resorption.[41]

Oral Malodor can also be found in cases of osteomyelitis, osteonecrosis, and malignancy.

EXTRA ORAL CAUSES OF HALITOSIS

The various systemic diseases capable of producing halitosis with the characteristics of the odor are described in **Table V.**[2]

Table V: Odorous Volatiles in The Breath Of Patients With Extraoral Blood-Borne Halitosis

Causes of blood-borne halitosis	Odorant
Systemic diseases	
Hepaticfailure/liver cirrhosis	Dimethylsulfide
Uremia/kidney failure	Dimethylamine, Trimethylamine Acetone
Diabetic ketoacidosis, diabetes mellitus	
Metabolic disorders	
Isolated persistent hypermethioninemia	Dimethylsulfide
Fish odor syndrome, trimethylaminuria	Trimethylamine
Medication	Carbon disulfide Dimethyl
Disulfiram	sulfide Dimethylsulfide
Dimethylsulfoxide	
Cysteamine	Allyl methylsulfide
Food Garlic	Methylpropylsulfide

Respiratory system

Post nasal drip is often associated with chronic sinusitis or regurgitation esophagitis, in which the acidic content of the stomach reaches the nasopharynx and causes mucositis. This rather common condition is perceived by the patients as a liquid flow in the throat originating from the oral cavity.[7] *Ozena* (caused by *Klebsillaozenae*) is a rare atrophic condition of the nasal mucosa with the appearance of crusts and causing a very strong breath malodor.[7] Pulmonary causes include chronic bronchitis, bronchiectasis (infection of standing mucus secretion in cystic dilations through walls of bronchioles), and bronchial carcinoma in which breath malodor is seen.[7] In acute rheumatic fever there is acid sweet odor. Foul putrefactive breath simulating odorous rotting meat is indicative of lung abscess or bronchiectasis.[42]

Chronic caseous tonsillitis (CCT) is frequently correlated to halitosis and is also a common disease. Palatine tonsils contain crypts that may retain exfoliated epithelium cells, keratin debris and foreign particles, forming a tonsillolith. Therefore, palatine tonsils are the most suitable sites for the activity of anaerobic bacteria in the upper airway system. Halitosis is one of the most common symptoms in patients with CCT and is present in about 77% of patients with CCT. The main causes of halitosis among CCT patients are related to decomposition of organic material such as food debris and putrefaction of amino acids by anaerobic proteolytic bacteria that increase the production of Volatile Sulfur Compounds in the tonsillary crypts. Clinically, these patients often describe worse halitosis symptoms when they expel a tonsillolith, but this has not yet been objectively documented. The presence of a tonsillolith therefore represents a ten fold risk factor for halitosis and is correlated to abnormal Volatile Sulfur Compounds halitometry in patients with CCT.[43]

Gastrointestinal tract

Helicobacter pylori is a spiral, microaerophilic, Gram negative bacterium that colonizes the human gastrointestinal tract, primarily the stomach. It is also believed to be responsible for gastritis and peptic ulcers, and is a risk factor for gastric cancer. Several studies have detected *H. pylori* in the human oral cavity, particularly in patients with gingivitis or chronic periodontitis, and have thus suggested that the oral cavity is the primary extra gastric reservoir for *H.pylori*. In contrast, other studies have failed to find evidence supporting the role of the oral cavity as a major reservoir of *H. pylori*. *H. pylori* has been suggested to have a special preference for the activated state of inflammation in periodontitis and several studies have reported that carriage of *H.pylori* may be associated with periodontal disease. The presence of *H. pylori* in the oral cavity may be related to halitosis through periodontal pocketing and inflammation, rather than Volatile Sulfur Compounds producing ability.[44]

Zenker's diverticulum can cause a significant breath odor because it is not separated from the oral cavity by any sphincter.[7] *Gastric hernia* (fundus of stomach protrudes through diaphragm with relative sphincter insufficiency, allowing gases to escape or contents to flow back in esophagus) can cause reflux of the gastric contents up to the oropharynx. This is sometimes concerned with rectus, where air from the stomach suddenly regurgitates.[7]

Hunger can give rise to oral malodor, and although there is little objective evidence to support this, this is common experience. The odor might be due to putrefaction of pancreatic juice in the stomach during hunger periods. Volatile Sulfur Compounds are reduced in the breath for 2 to 3 hour after a meal.[28]

Metabolic disorders (blood borne)

In cases of blood-borne halitosis' it is quite possible that virtually any odourous compound that satisfies the criteria of volatility, if generated within the body and having access to the bloodstream, could give rise to an oral malodour. Trimethylamine is such a compound. It is a simple tertiary aliphatic amine with a pungent ammonical odour approaching that of rotten fish at low concentrations and the human nose is extremely sensitive to this molecule, with some individuals being able to detect less than one part in 109. It is produced in excess in a metabolic disorder known as trimethylaminuria or the 'fish-odour syndrome'. Biochemically, the disorder is characterized by the presence of 'greater than normal' amounts of trimethylamine within the body. These high levels are present owing to a failure in removing the amine via the usual oxidation route to the non-odourous metabolite, trimethylamine N-oxide. This situation arises from a mismatch in the enzyme's capacity to undertake this metabolic reaction and the substrate load it has to process. Consequently, in principle, it appears that there are two major sub-types of the condition. Firstly, there are those forms that are related to a dysfunction of the normal enzyme activity owing to genetic, hormonal or inhibitory- chemical influences. Secondly, are those forms arising from substrate overload of the enzyme activity (normal or depressed) such as an excess of dietary precursors of trimethylamine or variations in gut microorganisms resulting in enhanced liberation of trimethylamine substrate. Clearly, these are two intimately related aspects. A substrate burden that is easily handled by one individual may become a substrate overload in another that has a decreased enzyme function for whatever reasons. Since the presence of excess trimethylamine depends upon interplay of numerous events, the odour problems associated with this condition usually vary in intensity and maybe transient in nature. When levels of trimethylamine are high, the volatile compound will leave the body via many routes (e.g. urine, sweat, breath, bodily secretions) best owing upon the patient an odourous aura resembling that of rotten or decaying fish. However, when the levels of trimethylamine are lower, then the odour may only be noticeable arising from freshly voided tepid urine or exhaled on the warm breath. This maybe particularly true for individuals who are heterozygous for the condition, in which free trimethylamine only approaches threshold levels when several factors unfortunately occur in concert.[45]

Acetone produces a sweet fruity odor which could indicate diabetic acidosis or impending hyperglycemic coma. Normal level of acetone in alveolar air is 1μg acetone/litre alveolar air. By measuring level of acetone in alveolar air, level of ketone bodies in arterial blood can be determined.[46] Type I (insulin dependent) diabetes in particular can result in the accumulation of ketones. The lack of glucose leads to breakdown of fat and proteins, resulting in ketone bodies such as acetoacetate and hydroxybutyrate. Type 2 (non insulin dependent) diabetes often remains undiagnosed for years; perception of breath malodor may provide a clue to its diagnosis.[7]

Liver

In patients with liver insufficiency, such as cirrhosis, ammonium will accumulate in the blood and will be exhaled.[7] The breath known as "fetor hepaticus" produces a sweetish, feculent, "amine odor" resembling a fresh cadaver. This kind of breath is often followed by hepatic coma. Sometimes such breath is also present in the patient with extensive portocavalvenous anastomoses, butitis by nature, intermittent for a long period of time.[7,47]

Kidney

Kidney insufficiency, primarily caused by chronic glomerulonephritis, will lead to an increased uric acid level in the blood, which is expressed in the expired air with a typical ammonium-like breath.[7]

Drugs (blood borne)

It is important to note that some medications for allergy and high blood pressure, antidepressants, and sinus medication can give rise to blood-borne halitosis. Metabolites of many drugs have been found to be excreted via the lungs. A good example is disulfiram (Antabuse), a drug used in treating alcoholism, which is metabolized to carbon disulfide. Antineoplastic medications may indirectly contribute to halitosis due to mucositis, ulceration, and increased gingival inflammation. Drugs associated with breath malodor are Tobacco, Alcohol, Chloral hydrate, Nitrites and nitrates, Dimethyl sulfoxide, Disulfiram, Cytotoxic agents, Phenothiazines, Amphetamines.[2]

Menstrual cycles

There is evidence on the influence of menstrual cycle and premenstrual syndrome on the production of Volatile Sulfur Compounds. Calil CM et al.[48] conducted a study on the influence of menstrual cycle and gender on the production of Volatile Sulfur Compounds and found higher levels of Volatile Sulfur Compounds in women during the premenstrual and menstrual phases when compared with the follicular phase and men. The lower Volatile Sulfur Compounds index found in men could be associated with androgens. A decreased salivary flow was observed during the premenstrual and menstrual phases. Reduced salivary flow weakens the normal cleansing mechanism of the mouth and could predispose the oral flora toward the Gram-negative organisms responsible for the malodor.

RELATIONSHIP BETWEEN ORAL MALODOR AND PERIDOONTAL DISEASE

Although tongue coating and periodontal conditions have been reported to be major halitosis-inducing factors,[2,6,50,51,52,53,54] the relationship between volatile sulfur compounds (VSC) and these two major factors is not yet fully understood.[52]

Halitosis has been reported to be caused by the same microorganisms causing gingivitis and periodontitis.

Three oral bacterial species highly associated with periodontal disease—*Porphyromonas gingivalis, Treponema denticola, and Tannerella forsythia* —are among the most active volatile sulfur compound producers in vitro. The presence of these organisms in dental plaque can be detected based on their ability to hydrolyze the synthetic trypsin substrate N-benzoyl-

DL-arginine-2-napthylamide (BANA).[50] It has been reported that the Volatile Sulfur Compound level and the Methyl Mercaptan / Hydrogen Sulfide ratio in mouth air from patients with periodontal involvement were 8 times higher than those of control subjects.[52] 4 times more tongue coating was found in patients with periodontitis than periodontally healthy controls.[52] Deep and inflamed crevicular sites exhibit a significantly higher Methyl Mercaptan/Hydrogen Sulfide ratio than the corresponding shallow or non-inflamed crevicular sites, and total sulfur in the deep and inflamed sites is significantly higher than in the corresponding shallow and non-inflamed sites.[52] It has also been proposed that the existence of active inflammation in periodontal tissue is more important than the mere presence of deeper periodontal pockets for the production of oral malodor.[52]

Studies have suggested that periodontitis increases the severity of oral malodor.[6] The bleeding tendency of the periodontal tissues may provide essential substrates for odor production.[6] The inflamed periodontal tissues provide more methionine, which is converted into methyl mercaptan at a higher rate than in healthy gingival tissues. The increased gingival crevicular fluid flow in periodontitis may be a continual source of methionine.[6] There is a correlation between Volatile Sulfur Compound in mouth air and the extent of periodontal disease, which implies that the Gram-negative anaerobic microflora, which increases in the subgingival plaque when there is periodontal inflammation, can contribute to these Volatile Sulfur Compound.[51] When subjects reporting oral malodor were studied, the BANA scores obtained from various loci (saliva, periodontal pockets, and tongue) were positively associated with oral malodor.[50]

The amount of tongue coating is closely correlated with oral malodor. The average amount of tongue coating is 6 times greater in individuals with periodontal disease. This coating is comprised of epithelial cells, leukocytes, and microorganisms released from periodontal pockets.[6] Tongue scraping of subjects with a high organoleptic score yielded more BANA (+) bacteria such as *Porphyromonas gingivalis*, *Bacteroides forsythus*, and *Treponema denticola*.[52] These results suggest that the interdental spaces in poor periodontal health contribute a higher proportion of all 3 Volatile Sulfur Compound productions than those with healthy periodontium.

Recent studies by Tsai C-C et al (2008),[53] Calil C et al

(2009)[54] show a weak association between Volatile Sulfur Compound and periodontal conditions (probing pocket depth, clinical attachment loss, gingival index).

TRANSITION FROM HEALTH TO GINGIVITIS

Gingivitis is characterized by an immune response to antigens in bacterial plaque as well as by alterations in connective tissue. One of the earliest events associated with disease is enhanced permeability of the lining epithelium within the gingival sulcus. Bacterial antigens such as lipopolysaccharide (LPS) induce gingival inflammation in some individuals but mere exposure to these antigens is not necessarily sufficient to cause gingivitis in all patients.

Volatile Sulfur Compounds are potentially capable of altering permeability of the gingival tissues, inducing inflammatory responses, and modulating functions of gingival fibroblasts **(Figure II).** Early work by Rizzo[55] indicated that a facilitating agent is required to allow LPS to penetrate healthy gingival epithelium and subsequently initiate an inflammatory response. Although no inflammatory response could be initiated by topical application of LPS to healthy gingiva, exposure of these tissues to H2S facilitated penetration of LPS and resulted in inflammation.

Figure II: Effects of Volatile Sulfur Compounds Which May Potentiate Gingivitis And Periodontitis Effect on Non-keratizinzed soft tissues

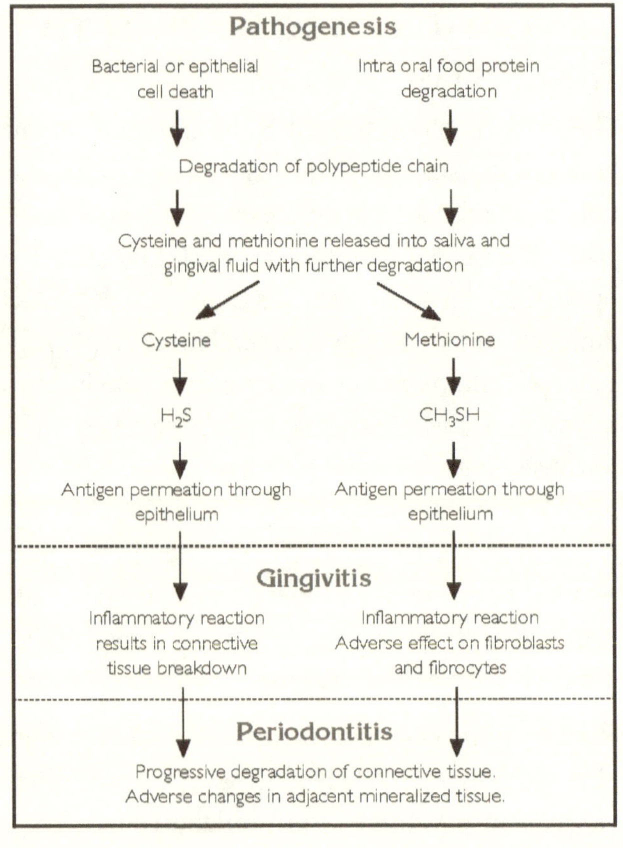

Ng and Tonzetich[56] demonstrated that not only Volatile Sulfur Compound can alter non-keratinized soft tissues, but also that these compounds can cause changes at low concentrations and within short periods of time. Also, Volatile Sulfur Compounds are not only directly toxic to tissues, but they may also facilitate entry of other bacterial antigens, such as LPS, into the underlying lamina propria. These data are consistent with the hypothesis that thiols participate in early stages of the inflammatory response and may be importantinitiators of gingivitis.

Methyl Mercaptan has been shown to induce secretion of interleukin-1 beta (IL-1ß) from mononuclear cells in culture. IL-1ß has been isolated from inflamed gingival tissue and may play a significant role in the pathogenesis of periodontal disease. Methyl mercaptan has also been shown to act synergistically with both LPS and IL-1ß to increase secretion of prostaglandin E2 and collagenase, important mediators of inflammation and tissue destruction. At present, the effects of Volatile Sulfur Compound on the physiology of blood vessels have not been studied and are an important area for future research.[29]

Effect on extracellular matrix formation

Volatile Sulfur Compound has direct effects on the formation of extracellular matrix by humangingival fibroblasts in culture. Experiments have demonstrated that exposure to either Hydrogen Sulfide or Methyl Mercaptan for between 24 and 48 hours lowers total protein production by these cells.[29] In addition, although both thiol compounds lower protein content, methyl mercaptan has the greater effect. Methyl mercaptan has been shown to inhibit synthesis of collagen as well. The concentrations of thiols employed (2ppm) were slightly higher than normally seen in mouth air of periodontal patients (0.5ppm). However, since concentrations detected in mouth air are diluted by ambient air, the higher amounts used are likely comparable to levels in periodontal pockets.[29]

Effects on collagen metabolism

The effects of Methyl Mercaptan on collagen metabolism are a reflection of both decreased synthesis and increased degradation of protein. Hydroxyproline analysis of mercaptan-exposed fibroblasts has demonstrated that both aspects of collagen metabolism are affected. In addition, the increased degradation is likely associated with inhibition of procollagen peptidase enzymes which are essential for procollagen processing since elevated amounts of procollagens can be demonstrated in Methyl Mercaptan-exposed gingival fibroblast cultures. Since procollagens will not efficiently cross-link and form mature collagen fibrils, these immature collagens are likely susceptible to enzymatic degradations. Inhibition of procollagen peptidases would therefore affect both synthesis and degradation of collagens. The effects of both Methyl Mercaptan and Hydrogen Sulfide on proteins likely result from the Inherent reactivity of the thiol (-SH) group in both of these compounds.[29] Previous studies with type I collagen have demonstrated that both of these gases, when labeled with radioactive sulfur, will bind to collagen and that a significant amount of the sulfur incorporated into the protein is tightly bound (likely through covalent binding). Dimethyl disulfide, a Volatile Sulfur Compound which does not have a reactive thiol, is essentially inert.[29]

THE TRANSITION FROM GINGIVITIS TO PERIODONTITIS

In the change from gingivitis to periodontitis, there is a continuation of all the events in the oral malodor and gingivitis sections as well as a new group of events that occur in the development of periodontitis. Periodontitis results from destruction of both the hard and soft tissue structures which support teeth. The transition from gingivitis to periodontitis is mainly an anatomical difference in which the disease progresses into the underlying bone.[29]

Effect on periodontal ligament

Since the periodontal ligament (PDL) is associated with the formation and maintenance of the mineralized supporting structures, effects of thiols on these ligament cells are particularly relevant. Moreover, since the major extracellular matrix (ECM) protein in bone is type I collagen, alterations in collagen will likely have a dramatic effect on hard tissues. Experiments which have correlated increases in periodontal probing depth and bleeding on probing with increases in methyl mercaptan in these pockets are also relevant since they indicate that effects resulting from exposure to Methyl Mercaptan become increasingly important in periodontitis.[29] These observations are in accordance with results obtained from analysis of mouth air of periodontal patients which have demonstrated a correlation between increases in Methyl Mercaptan / Hydrogen Sulfide concentration ratios and increases in periodontal pocket depth.

Studies have shown that periodontal ligament cells exposed to methyl mercaptan in culture alter their intracellular pH and become more acidic. In addition, they exhibit decreased motility, lowered protein synthesis, and alterations in collagen metabolism. These changes are predominantly detrimental to the ability of these cells to maintain or regenerate mineralized tissues. Results have indicated that exposure of PDL cells to Methyl Mercaptan results in changes in collagens which are much like those observed in gingival fibroblasts exposed to mercaptan. There appears to be a similar inhibition of procollagen peptidases resulting in accumulation of procollagen precursors. In addition, there are substantial reductions in amounts of type III collagens. This observation is significant since periodontally involved tissues are known to exhibit substantial losses of type III collagens which decrease from 20 - 30% to 4% of total collagens.[29]

Other ECM proteins are also affected. Fibronectin in periodontal cell cultures treated with mercaptan exhibits less disulfide-mediated cross-linking. These cells, rather than producing high-molecular weight multimers, produce fibronectin of lower molecular weight which corresponds to monomeric rather than the usual dimeric or multimeric protein. Since both collagen and fibronectin play important roles in cell migration, changes in these ECM molecules may contribute to the decreases in cell motility observed in periodontal cell cultures exposed to Methyl Mercaptan.[29]

Effect on alveolar bone

Volatile Sulfur Compounds might be one of the pathogenic factors causing alveolar bone loss in periodontitis.[57] The gingival sulcular epithelium has an important role in inhibiting the invasion of microbial products in the gingival sulcus. That is, the gingival sulcular epithelium is a barrier preventing periodontal conditions. It has been suggested that Volatile Sulfur Compounds may decrease the barrier effect of the gingival sulcular epithelium, as Volatile Sulfur Compound inhibit the growth or proliferation of human gingival epithelial cells.[57] Hydrogen Sulfide penetrates though the entire tissue layers of the gingival crevicular mucosa model. These results indicate that the toxic effects of Hydrogen Sulfide may even occur in the alveolar bone. According to a study conducted by Imai T et al.[57] Hydrogen Sulfide was shown to inhibit the proliferation of normal human osteoblast and murine osteoblastic cell line (MC3T3-E1) in a dose-dependent manner. Volatile Sulfur Compounds, such as Hydrogen Sulfide, produced by oral microorganisms might be a causative factor of alveolar bone absorption.

DIAGNOSIS

An average person can detect unpleasant smell, and almost everyone has some experience of bad breath in others. Clinical research on halitosis requires more than just detection of odour; odour needs to be quantified. Unlike quantification of intensities of light, sound, smoke or heat, quantification of odour sensation is very difficult; and even more difficult is the controlled presentation of odour to stimulate its perception by the odour judges. Another difficulty in odour research is that once a halitosis patient expels breath for estimation by one judge, the odoriferous compound released subsequently for other judges may differ in composition and intensity. Despite these difficulties our knowledge of halitosis has increased owing to a better understanding of its aetiology and improved methods of collecting and analyzing odoriferous compounds.[5]

CLINICAL EVALUATION AND ORAL EXAMINATION

In practice, the flowchart in **Figure III** is suggested for patients with complaints of halitosis.[2] Before the first appointment all patients receive detailed medical and halitosis questionnaires as well as written instructions. The general medical questionnaire, which includes questions about e.g. systemic diseases, allergy, asthma, rhinitis, sinusitis, and medication, has to be filled in before the appointment and can be discussed beforehand with the physician if needed. Additionally a specific halitosis questionnaire is given to the patient. It is important to start the examination by firstly carrying out both subjective and objective assessment of the degree of halitosis and then start the intraoral examination. In this way, the severity of the halitosis is assessed before any changes in the degree of halitosis can occur. During the first visit, extensive of soft tissue, hard tissue, and periodontal examinations are performed in order to determine whether the patient has other oral health problems.

Specific attention is paid to the tongue and the presence of tongue debris is noted using a tongue coating index.

Figure III: Flow Chart in Halitosis Practice

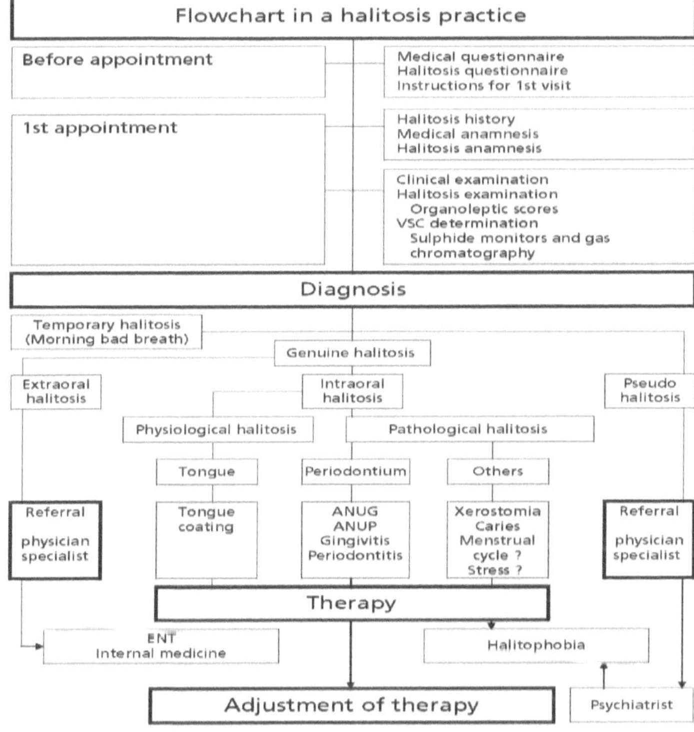

INDEX SYSTEMS FOR TONGUE COATING

The tongue is normally pink but a very thin whitish coating can also be considered normal. Having a coating on the tongue does not necessarily mean that bad breath is present, although heavy tongue coatings are usually positively related to halitosis. Various index systems developed over the years are as follows.

Miyazaki et al.[58] divides the tongue into three sections and the presence or absence of tongue coating is registered as follows:

score 0 = none visible;

score 1 = less than one third of tongue dorsum is covered;

score 2 = between one and two thirds;

score 3 = more than two thirds.

Gomez et al.[59] divides the tongue into nine different sections, whilst Winkel et al.[60] divides the tongue into six sections, three in the posterior and three in the anterior part of the tongue. Each sextant is categorized as:

score 0 = no coating present;

score 1 = presence of a light coating;

score 2 = presence of a distinct coating.

The resulting Winkel tongue coating index (WTCI) is obtained by adding all six scores.[60] **(Figure IV)**

FIGURE IV: Winkel Tongue Coating Index

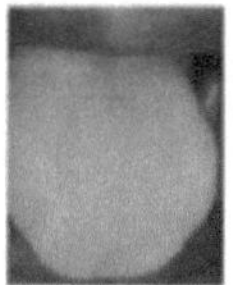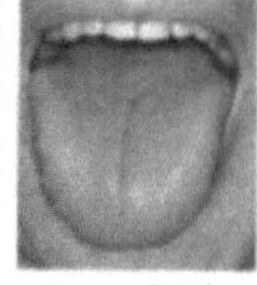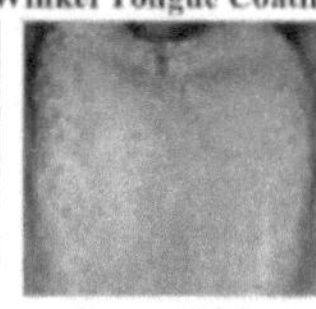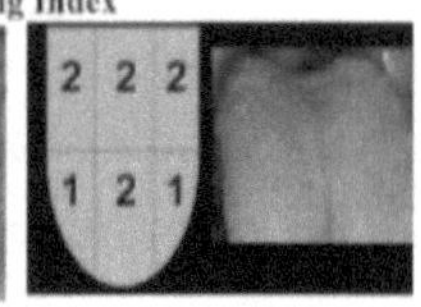

| Normal Tongue (Without Coating) | Tongue With Light Coating | Tongue With Heavy Coating | Winkel Tongue Coating Index (WTCI) |

MEASUREMENT METHODS OF HALITOSIS:

The three primary measurement methods of genuine halitosis are:
1. Organoleptic measurement,
2. Gas chromatography, and
3. Sulphide monitoring.

Additional or alternative measurement methods are:

4. BANA test,
5. Chemical sensors,
6. Quantifying β-galactosidase activity,
7. Salivary incubation test,
8. Ammonia monitoring,
9. Ninhydrin method,
10. Polymerase chain reaction,
11. Tongue Sulfide Probe,
12. Zinc Oxide Thin Film Conductor Sensor,
13. OraTest, and
14. Self Assessment of Oral Malodor

1) Organoleptic measurement (Figure V)

Organoleptic orhedonic measurement is a simple commonly used measurement method of halitosis by an examiner.

Odor Judges:

Before acting as a judge, persons must ensure they do not have anosmia (lost or impaired smelling capacity). A significant fraction of the adult population has partial loss of smelling acuity. After age 60, a decline of smelling acuity is common. Candidate odor judges should test their capacity to smell and recognize different odors (qualitative assessment) as well as their capacity to detect odors at low concentrations (quantitative assessment). The first aspect can be checked by using commercially available tests (smell identification test, Sensonic) that establishes a response curve based on the capacity to recognize and discriminate among smells.

After scratching an odorous surface in a booklet, several options of smells are proposed. If a subject lacks the capacity to recognize certain odors, it will reveal a partial anosmia. The second aspect is tested by sniffing a series of dilutions of substances, such as isovaleric acid, phenethyl alcohol, thiophene, and pyridine, which are in expensive organic components. These are presented to the candidate judge as dilutions, in on-log dilution steps, from 1 to 10^{-19}. Concentrations of the odorous substance are presented in ascending order until the subject detects the substance, then in descending order until the person no longer detects it. This is the "psychophysical staircase method" for determination of the threshold level. The threshold corresponds to the average between ascending and descending levels. Clinicians must find out if their smelling threshold level is normal. Abnormalities in the capacity to judge or perceive odors can be caused by a viral infection of the nasal cavities, a concussion, and smoking. Whereas infection can have transient effects on olfactory performance, concussion and smoking have permanent effects.[7] Agreement among judges maybe increased by standardization of the sense of smell, using an odour solution kit for measuring the olfactory sense and previously assigned scores. The use of n-butanol as a suitable odorant for use in organoleptic training of breath odour judges cannot be assessed as a helpful method. The scores did not correlate with gas chromatography scores at all and the use of n-butanol can not be recommended because of its irritant nature.[3] In a study it was seen that the percentage of agreement in scores between organoleptic judges exceeded 83%.[61] It was also seen that sensory training exercises reduced oral judges' errors.[62]

Method:

Patients are instructed to abstain from taking antibiotics for three weeks before the assessment, to abstain from eating garlic, onion and spicy foods for 48 hours before the assessment and to avoid using scented cosmetics for 24 hours before the assessment. Patients are instructed to abstain from ingesting any food or drink, to omit their usual oral hygiene practices, to abstain from using oral rinse and breath fresheners, and to abstain from smoking for 12 hours before the assessment. The oral malodor examiner, who should have a normal sense of smell, is required to refrain from drinking coffee, tea or juice, and to refrain from smoking and using scented cosmetics before the assessment.[34]

A plastic tube is inserted into the patient's mouth, preventing the dilution of mouth air with room air. While the patient is exhaling slowly, the examiner judges the odour at the other end of the tube. A privacy screen with a hole for the straw or the tube can be used to separate the examiner from the patient. Nasal-breath odour can be measured with a tube inserted into one of the nostrils, while the other nostril is closed by a finger.

Various scoring systems can be used for estimating the intensity of the odour. The most widely used scale is ranging from 0 to 5:

0 = no odour,

1= barely noticeable odour,

2 = slight but clearly noticeable odour,

3 = moderate odour,

4 = strong odour,

5 = extremely foul odour.

FIGURE V: Steps in Organoleptic Measurement

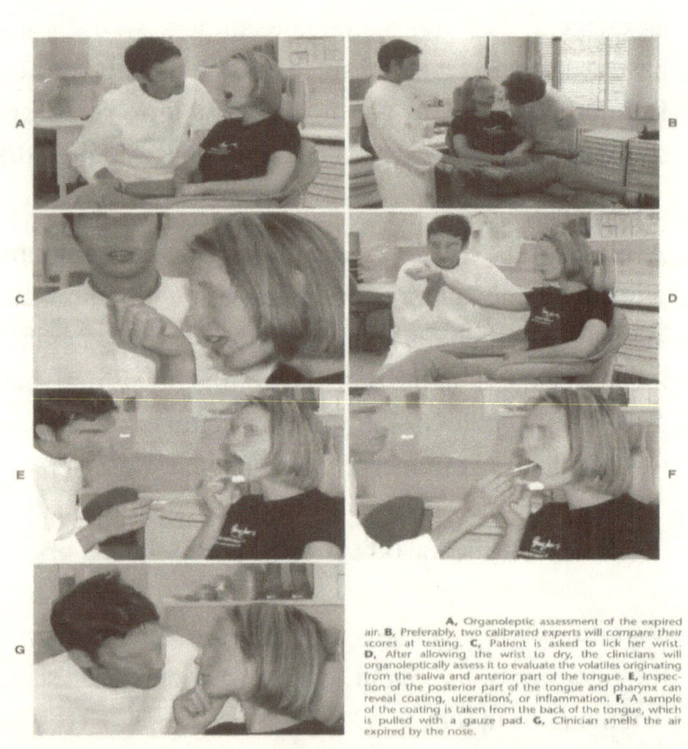

A, Organoleptic assessment of the expired air. B, Preferably, two calibrated experts will compare their scores at testing. C, Patient is asked to lick her wrist. D, After allowing the wrist to dry, the clinicians will organoleptically assess it to evaluate the volatiles originating from the saliva and anterior part of the tongue. E, Inspection of the posterior part of the tongue and pharynx can reveal coating, ulcerations, or inflammation. F, A sample of the coating is taken from the back of the tongue, which is pulled with a gauze pad. G, Clinician smells the air expired by the nose.

The judge smells a series of different air samples, as follows:[7]

1. *Oral cavity odor*: the subject opens the mouth and refrains from breathing while the judge places his or her nose close to the mouth opening. (Smelling the air while patient counts from 1 to 20 reveals the same but favors oral malodor because drying of the palatal and tongue mucosa will occur, which promotes the expression of Volatile Sulfur Compounds thus far soluble in salivary coating.)
2. *Breath odor*: the subject expires air through the mouth while the judge smells both at the beginning (determined by the oral cavity and systemic factors) and at the end (originating from the bronchi and lungs) of the expiration.
3. *Tongue coating*: the judge smells a tongue scraping. This is also presented to the patient or the confidant to evaluate whether this smell is similar to the experienced malodor.
4. *Nasal breath odor*: the subject expires through the nose, keeping the mouth closed. When the nasal expiration is malodorous, whereas the air expired through the mouth is not, a nasal/paranasal cause is suspected.

Disadvantages of organoleptic method:

- Although a good correlation between Volatile Sulfur Compounds concentration and organoleptic values has been found, it is still a subjective test, and when the examiners are repeatedly exposed to bad odors they become adapted to them and lose sensitivity.
- Dentists, especially periodontists, may not be ideal judges if they do not use masks on a regular basis.
- There is also the potential risk of disease transmission to the examiner through the expelled air. This is particularly important with the existence of epidemic bird flu infections and other acute respiratory illnesses.[5]

<u>Newer Developments</u> (Figure VI)

A possible solution to overcome these limitations is to use a more systemized and standardized method of organoleptic testing for measuring halitosis. One of this method is ***Kim organoleptic method,***[63] which uses a gas tight syringe and a paper cup connected to a plastic straw to measure halitosis.

Figure VI: Organoleptic Measurement by the New Organoleptic Method

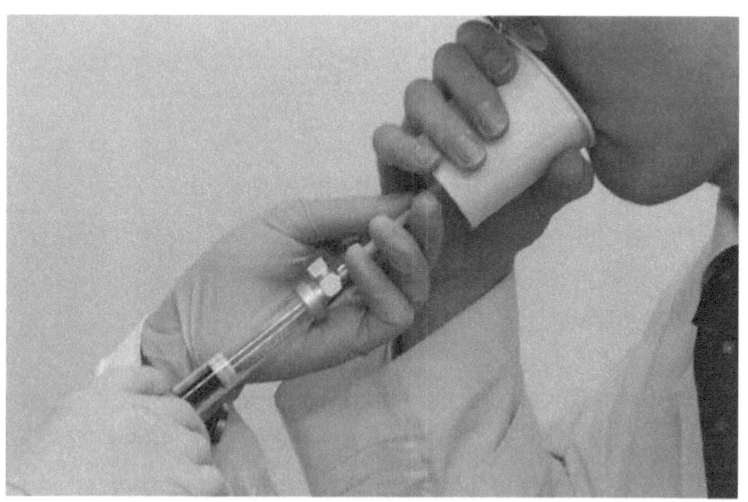

Method:

A disposable paper cup is used to perform the organoleptic test. A small hole is made at the base of the cup to insert a disposable 6.5mm plastic straw. A thin wax film is used to seal the connection. For a more precise organoleptic test, one examiner should place the cup over his nose, and another examiner expell the sample through the plastic tube into the cup. All organoleptic scores are assigned by one examiner.

The organoleptic rating is estimated on a scale of 0 to 4 as described by De Boever and Loesche[47] as described below:

0 = no appreciable odor;

1. =barely noticeable odor that is of low intensity and with inacceptable limits;

2. = slight to moderate odor that is clearly noticeable and slightly unpleasant;

3. =moderate to high odor that is clearly noticeable, unpleasant, and of moderate intensity, and

4. = offensive odor of strong intensity.

Advantages:

- The subject is prevented from observing the direct sniffing procedure of the examiner, the oral air samples can be separated from the subjects, and low concentrations of gases can be detected.
- The use of a gas tight syringe leads the patient to believe that one is the subject of a specific malodor examination rather than the direct-sniffing procedure.
- It is possible to obtain halitosis samples that are not diluted by room air that originates from the peri-oral region.

The ***spoon test***[6] is a simple, all be it subjective, organoleptic measurement method. Using a spoon or similar instrument, the tongue dorsum is scraped and the scraped material can be smelled.

2) Gas chromatography (Figure VII)

Quantitative analysis of Volatile Sulfur Compounds by a gas chromatography (GC) equipped with a flame photometric detector (FPD) is considered one of the most reliable measurements for diagnosing halitosis. With gas chromatography the concentration of volatile sulphur-containing compounds in samples of saliva, tongue coating or expired breath is measured by producing mass spectra. Samples are analyzed by a gas chromatograph equipped with a flame photometric detector.

The components can be identified by comparing the mass spectra with those of a computer based reference library. Gas Chromatography maybe combined with mass spectrometry, enlarging the scope of the method.[3]

Figure VII: Gas chromatograph with flame photometric detector (Trade name: Reconditioned Perkin Elmer Autosystem Xl Gc)[TM]

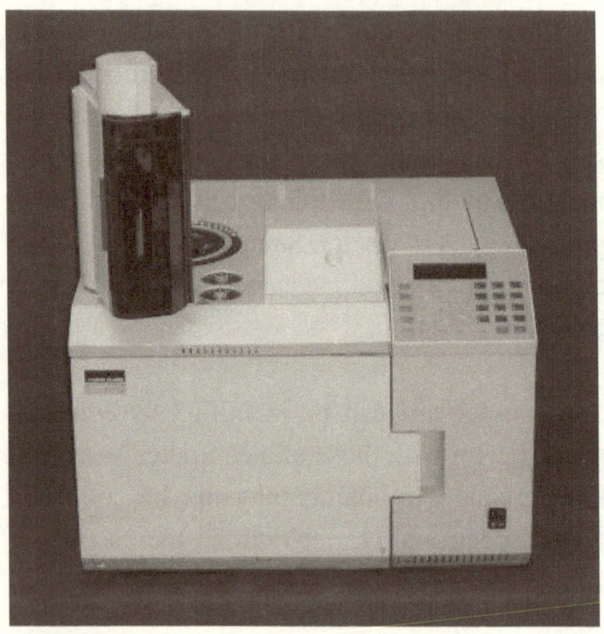

Advantages:

- GC-FPD measurement is very dependable because of its specificity to volatile sulfur compounds; the Gas Chromatography method is originally highly objective and reproducible.

Disadvantages:

- GC-FPD is a sophisticated piece of equipment that requires an experienced operator.

- The device is costly and very large. Therefore, it is impractical to use it for routine examinations in dental practices.[8]

Newer Developments (FIGURE VIII)

A compact and simple Gas Chromatography equipped with a newly invented ***indium oxide (In2O3) semiconductor gas sensor (SCS),***[8] which is highly sensitive to all kinds of volatile sulfur compounds has been developed recently. GC-SCS measures each Volatile Sulfur Compounds separately, whereas other devices cannot detect each separately.

Method:

For sampling, a three-way stopcock is incorporated between a 20-cm length of polytetra fluoro ethylene (PTFE) sampling tube (3.3-mm outside diameter) and the GC- FPD, and a 1ml disposable syringe was connected to the other arm of a three-way stopcock. Before each analysis, subjects are instructed to keep their mouths closed and to breathe through the nose for 30 seconds. The sampling tube is inserted into the center of the oral cavity through the lips and teeth, and the lips remained closed around it. After making sure saliva did not enter the tube, 15 ml oral air is aspirated with a gas-tight syringe connected to the outlet of the auto injector of the GC-FPD. A 10ml sample of the air is automatically transferred into the GC-FPD column and chromatographed. Immediately after aspirating 15ml oral air into the auto injector, 1ml oral air is aspirated twice by the syringe. Because of the dead-space effect in the syringe, the first aspirated sample is abandoned; and 0.5ml oral air from the second sample was injected into the GC-SCS. A single trained examiner performs all measurements for each gas chromatograph to avoid inter operator variation.[8]

Advantages:
- The cost of GC-SCS is 15% to 25% of a conventional GC-FPD.
- GC-SCS does not require hydrogen and carrier gas, which are essential for GC-FPD.
- The method is considered to be highly objective, reproducible, and reliable.

Disadvantages:

- It cannot be easily clinically implemented because of the relatively high cost, the requirement of highly trained persons, and the extensive procedures.

Figure VIII: GC-SCS and Sampling System

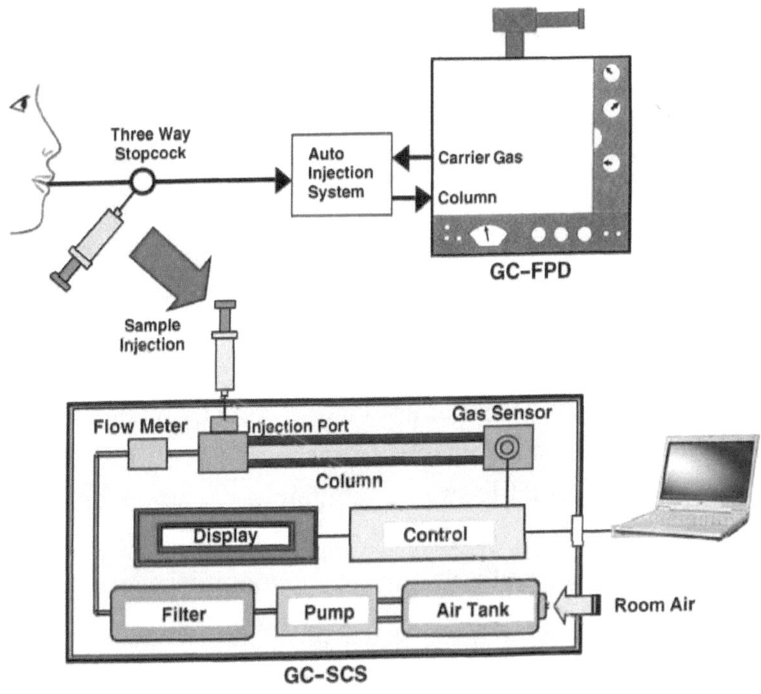

Newer Methods:

To eliminate discrepancies caused by variations in operator sampling or breath injection techniques, an automated system aspirating breath samples directly into the gas chromatograph was developed. In order to overcome the practical drawbacks, portable gas chromatographs were developed to measure Sulphur containing compound levels inside the mouth.[8]

3) Sulphide monitoring

Method:

Patients are asked to refrain from talking 5min prior to measurement. The monitor is zeroed on ambient air. Measurement is performed by inserting a disposable tube into the patient's mouth and connecting this to the monitor, while the patient is breathing through the nose. Electrochemical reactions with the sulphur-containing compounds in the breath generate an electric current, which is directly proportional to the levels of volatile sulphur-containing compounds.

Trade Names of portable sulfide monitors:

I)   *Halimeter* (Rosenberg et al.)[64]

II)   *Oral Chroma* (Miyazaki)[65]

III) *Breathtron* (Sopapornamorn)[66]

I) Halimeter (Interscan, US) **(Figure IX)**

The Halimeter device detects the presence of volatile sulfur compounds that are known to produce undesirable odours. Several readings are taken from are as such as the front of the mouth, the back of the mouth and the nostrils.

Figure IX: Halimeter (Interscan Corporation)

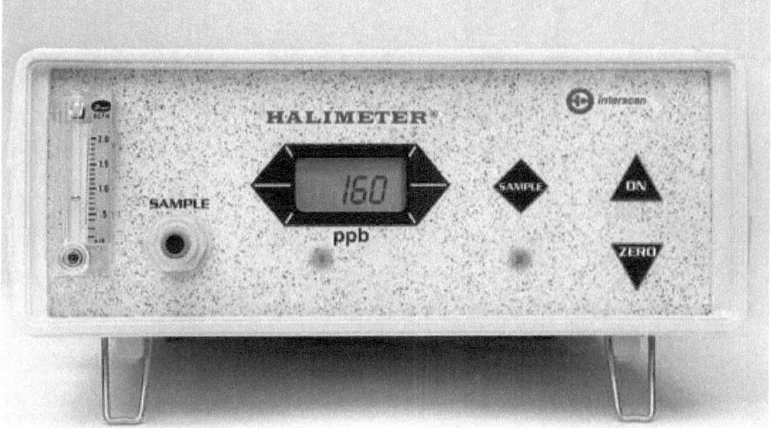

Sampling Technique:

The manner in which the sample is collected is critical to obtaining accurate readings. The proper sampling technique is described in detail below.

1. Ensure that the sample straw is inserted fully into the sample tube connector until it reaches the tubestop. If not fully inserted, sample may be lost to leakage at the connector.
2. The patient's mouth should remain closed for 3

minutes prior to sampling to allow a full build up of any volatile sulfur compounds present in the breath sample.

3. When ready to collect sample, the end of the sample straw should be inserted into the patient's mouth at a depth of approximately 1-2 inches (25-50mm) resting on the back of the tongue. The lips should be almost closed allowing for a slight gap between the lips and the sample straw. Do not press the lips or teeth down on the sample straw. Breathing should continue through the nose during sampling allowing sample to be drawn from the mouth into the Halimeter by the pump rather than forced in by the lungs.

4. Do not blow into the sample straw asthis will affect sample accuracy. The flow indicator should be monitored by the individual supervising the breath test to ensure that the flow rate stays at approximately 1.0 Standard Cubic Feet Per Hour (SCFH) and that it is not increasing or fluctuating as a result of the patient breathing or blowing into the sample straw.

5. Typically, the parts per billion (ppb) level will rise during the sample period and reach a peak value after which the value will beg into fall. When the sample parts per billion value begins to decrease, the sample straw should be removed from the mouth and set down until the next sample period at

which point the sequence will be repeated.[64]

Disadvantages:
- The Halimeter is unsuitable for measuring patients with extraoral halitosis from dimethyl sulfide.
- The Halimeter has a high sensitivity for hydrogen sulfide but a lower sensitivity for methyl mercaptan, which isa significant contributor to halitosis.
- Certain foods such as garlic and onions produce sulfur in the breath for as long as 48 hours and may result in false readings.
- The Halimeter is also very sensitive to alcohol, so one should avoid drinking alcohol or using alcohol containing mouthwashes for at least 12 hours prior to being tested.

II) <u>Oral Chroma (Abimedical Corporation)</u> (Figure X, XI)

Oral Chroma analyses the volatile sulfur compounds typically comprising halitosis, measures the individual concentrations of hydrogen sulfide, methyl mercaptan and dimethyl sulfide, and displays the concentrations on a display panel. Each of the three component gases, and the measured concentrations, can be correlated with a specific cause of halitosis.[65]

Figure X: Oral Chroma (Abimedical Corporation)

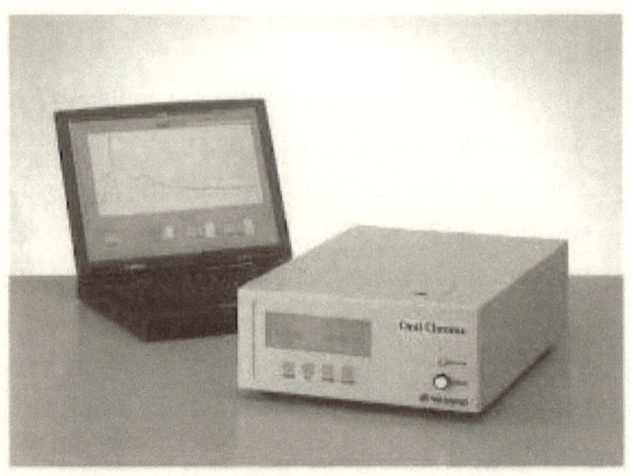

Figure XI: Three-Step Measuring Procedure by Oral Chroma

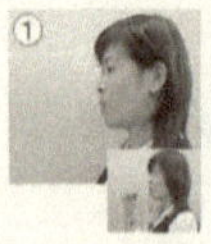

Insert the plastic syringe that comes with the product deep into the oral cavity and hold it between the lips. (Be careful to avoid touching the tongue with the syringe.) Then, slowly pull the plunger, push it in again, and pull it for the second time before removing the syringe from the mouth.

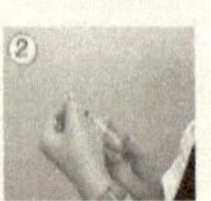

If the top of the syringe is wet, wipe it dry with a tissue.
Attach the dedicated needle and eject the sampled oral gas to 0.5 cc (1/2 calibration) by pushing the plunger.

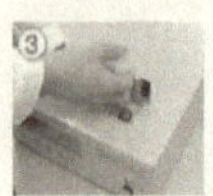

Inject the remaining oral gas into the inlet on the main unit of the OralChroma™. The measurement will now start automatically.

III)Breathtron (Yoshida, Tokyo, Japan) **(Figure XII)**

It is a semiconductor type sulfide monitor, which is composed of an air intake, sensor detector, control panel, digital display and printer. The semi-conductor sensor is based on a thick Zinc Oxide (ZnO) membrane that has a high specificity for Volatile Sulfur Compounds.

Figure XII: Breathtron (Yoshida Corporation)

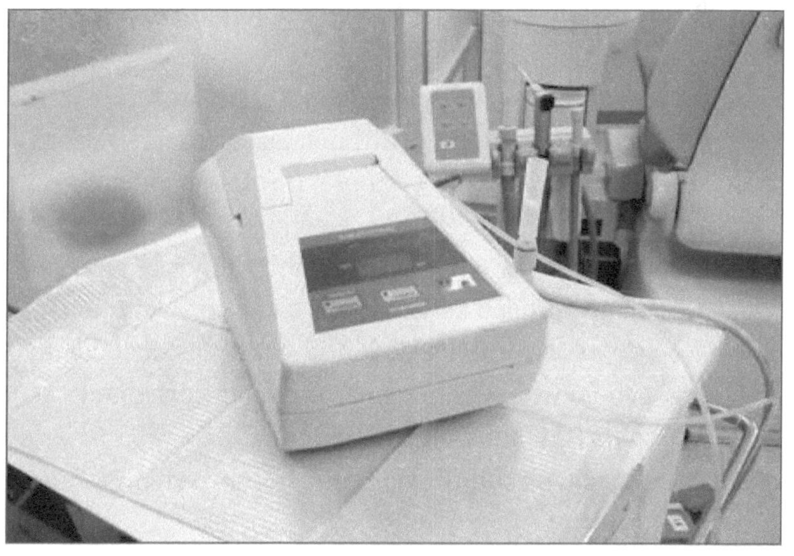

Method:

The disposable mouthpiece, which has a build-in filter to eliminate other volatile compounds (like ketone and alcohol in toothpaste and mouth wash), is inserted into an end of the Teflon tube connected to the monitor inlet. Breathtron requires 1 min an 45 sec for warm-up before operation, 45 sec for measurement and 1 min and 30 sec for each succeeding measurement. Measurements are performed by directly inserting the disposable mouthpiece into the patient's oral cavity. The patients are instructed to close their mouth tightly and breathe through their nose during the measurement. The aspiration rate of mouth air is 40–60ml per minute, and the Breathtron values are presented in units of parts per billion (ppb).[66]

Disadvantages of sulfide monitors:
- They are unable to differentiate between various sulfides. Because of this monitor's problem with differentiating sulfide compounds and because methyl mercaptan is three times more unpleasant than hydrogen sulfide at the same concentration, it is possible that it underestimates the malodor in people with high methyl mercaptan concentrations in their mouths.
- Results of sulfide monitors are interfered by high levels of ethanol or essential oils.
- Instrument sensitivity decreases over time that necessitates periodic recalibration.[10]

Sulphide monitor measurements correlated

significantly for mainly low correlation coefficients with organoleptic scores. Patients may produce normal sulphide monitor measurements, whereas organoleptic scores are high. The reason for this discrepancy is that in addition to volatile sulphide-containing compounds other odorants contribute to halitosis, such as volatile short-chain fatty acids, polyamines, alcohols, phenyl compounds, alkanes, ketones, and nitrogen-containing compounds. These odorants are not detectable by a sulphide monitor.[10]

Although several studies demonstrated thatgas chromatography and sulphide monitor measurements are highly significant correlated, appreciable differences were observed.[3] The sensitivity and specificity of gas chromatography (0.79 and 0.83, respectively) appeared higher than the sensitivity and specificity of sulphide monitoring (0.76 and 0.78, respectively). When relatively precise measurements are required, gas chromatography is the preferable method.

Newer Methods:

Recently, a new sulphide monitor was developed.[10] The monitor's sensitivity and specificity was, respectively, more than 0.79 and between 0.61 and 0.73. Because this monitor has a low specificity in periodontal disease patients, it should be used cautiously for measuring volatile sulphur-containing compounds related to periodontal disease.

4) BANA test (Figure XIII)

It is a chair side test that is used to determine the proteolytic activity of certain oral anaerobes that contribute to oral malodor. Proteolytic obligate Gram-negative anaerobes and short-chain fatty acids colonizing the subgingival plaque and the dorsum of the tongue can be detected by the presence of an enzyme degrading benzoyl-DL-arginine-a-naphthylamide (BANA), a synthetic trypsin substrate, and forming a colored compound. The name of the halitosis measurement method is BANA test.

Figure XIII: Bana Test Strips

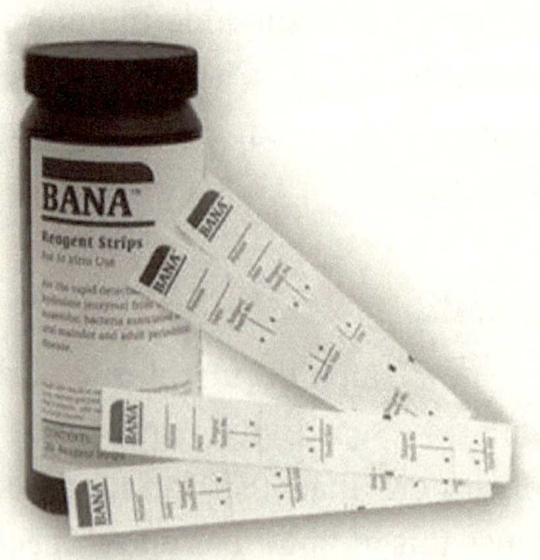

Method:

This test consists of incubating samples from plaque or the tongue with N benzoyl-DL-arginine-a-naphthylamide or BANA, which is a synthetic trypsin substrate. If the organisms have enzymes that degrade BANA, a colored compound is produced within roughly five to 15 minutes that indicates a positive BANA test. When patients are treated successfully to reduce and/or eliminate oral malodor, the tongue BANA test converts from positive to negative.[10]

Advantages:

The BANA test is a very practical and easy to use method.

Disadvantages:[67]

- It cannot determine the specific role of the different bacterial species in the production of halitosis.
- It only detects a limited number of pathogens.
- Does not include inhibitor of host protease which could contaminate the plaque sample for saliva, GCF and which also cleans BANA substrate.

Using a step-wise multiple regression analysis technique that combines a positive BANA test with Halimeter readings vastly improves the correlation of the combined readings with organoleptic scores.

BANA scores correlated significantly with organoleptic measurements, but were poorly related to sulphide monitor measurements. Probably, micro-organisms associated with BANA assay contribute malodorous components to the breath air other than sulphur-containing compounds, such as cadaverine.

In patients with periodontal disease, a stronger correlation between BANA test and sulphide monitor measurements was found.

5) Chemical sensors

Chemical sensors for volatile sulphur-containing compounds have been integrated into a probe for measuring directly in periodontal pockets and on the tongue. A sulphide-sensing element in the probe generates an electrochemical voltage proportional to the concentration of sulphide ions present. This voltage is measured relative to the operating point of a reference element. The electrochemical voltages generated by sulphide ions are measured by an electronic unit and displayed in a digital score. Measurements by a monitor with a zinc-oxide, thin film, and semiconductor sensor demonstrated highly significant correlations with organoleptic measurements.

<u>Electronic Nose[3]</u>

The *Electronic Nose* technique has recently been introduced, but the equipment is extremely costly.

Advantages:
- Electronic nose system can also detect such volatile compounds as organic compounds, aromatic compounds, amine-containing compounds, and ammonia derivatives in food and beverages. High correlations have been found with organoleptic as well as gas chromatography measurements.[3]

Disadvantages:

- A traditional problem with the use of electronic noses is the influence of water vapor.[68]
- This technique cannot determine volatile chemicals precisely, and it is difficult to distinguish mouth-air compounds from others present using this equipment.
- The mouth-air sample will be contaminated with a certain amount of respiratory air by this sampling procedure.[66]

Newer Developments:

Other promising chemical sensors for measuring ammonia and methyl mercaptan in breath air have been introduced lately.[3] Recently, a compact gas chromatograph with an indium oxide semiconductor gas sensor was developed. The apparatus measures each volatile sulphur-containing compound separately. Strong measurement correlations have been demonstrated between this apparatus and a conventional gas chromatograph.

6) Quantifying β-galactosidase activity

Deglycosylation of glycoproteins is considered as an initial step in oral malodour production. β-*Galactosidase* is one of the important enzymes in deglycosylation. The activity of β galactosidase can be easily quantified with the use of a chromogenic substrate absorbed onto a chromatography paper disc. Saliva applied to the paper disc, may induce a colour change of the paper, which can be recorded by an examiner:

0 = no colour;

1 = faint blue colour;

2 = moderate to dark blue colour.

β-Galactosidase assay scores were significantly associated with organoleptic scores for whole-mouth and tongue malodour (r = 0.47–0.49; p < 0.001). β-Galactosidase activity and sulphide monitor measurements both factored significantly into multiple regression equations for organoleptic scores, yielding multiple r-values ranging from 0.47 (p = 0.0007) to 0.60 (p < 0.0001)[3].

7) Salivary incubation test

Saliva is believed to be one of the main sources of oral malodor because it contains a large reservoir of sulphur-containing substrates that can be hydrolyzed and further degraded to volatile sulphur compounds. Therefore, salivary samples may be used for an indirect malodor examination.[69]

Method:

The salivary incubation test uses saliva collected in a glass tube. After incubating the tube at $37.8^{\circ}C$ in anaerobic chamber under an atmosphere of 80% nitrogen, 10% carbon dioxide, and 10% hydrogen for several hours, the odour can be measured by an examiner.

Advantages:

The salivary incubation test is much less influenced by external parameters, such as subjectivity, smoking, drinking coffee, eating garlic, onion, spicy food, and scented cosmetics, than organoleptic measurements.[3]

In a pilot study done by Quirynen M et al (2003)[69] for the evaluation of oral malodor by an in vitro salivary incubation test a strong correlation between the salivary incubation test and organoleptic as well as sulphide monitor measurements was demonstrated. In this immediately after breath assessments, 1.5 ml of unstimulated saliva was collected and equally divided into 3 sterile glass test tubes (15.5cm in length, diameter 1.5cm). These test tubes were then flushed with Carbon Dioxide and sealed with a rubber cup and tape. One tube was immediately reopened to measure the Volatile Sulfur Compounds (baseline value). The two remaining tubes were incubated at 37°C in an anaerobic chamber under an atmosphere of 80% nitrogen, 10% carbon dioxide, and 10% hydrogen, for 3 and 6 hours, respectively. Immediately after removal from the chamber, the odor of each tube was assessed both organoleptically and via the sulphide monitor. For the organoleptic ratings, the evaluator sniffed the head space air of the tubes and rated the smell as described above. The Volatile Sulfur Compounds levels were measured with the same portable sulphide monitor as used in a clinic, zeroed on ambient air prior to each measurement.

A disposable plastic straw was inserted 5cm into the tube. The peak Volatile Sulfur Compounds score was determined in parts per billion sulphur equivalents.

8) Ammonia monitoring

A portable monitor for measuring ammonia has been developed on the basis of the hypothesis that ammonia produced by oral bacteria reflects halitosis

Method:
Patients are instructed to rinse with a urea solution for 30s and to then keep their mouth closed for 5 min. The instrument contains a pump, which can draw air through an ammonia gas detector tube connected to a disposable mouthpiece placed inside a patient's mouth. The concentrations of ammonia produced by oral bacteria can be read directly from a scale.

Levels of volatile sulphur-containing compounds and ammonia were determined in 25 patients by gas chromatography and ammonia monitoring. A significant correlation existed between the two measurement methods. Bacteria in dental plaque and tongue coating produced ammonia in a concentration dependent manner. The ammonia level decreased after the removal of tongue coating and dental plaque.[3]

9) Ninhydrin method

Amines or polyamines cannot be measured by using sulphide monitoring. In a recent study, the ninhydrin method was used for detecting low-molecular-weight amines in breath.[3]

Method:

A sample of saliva and isopropanol is mixed and centrifuged. The supernatant is diluted with isopropanol, buffer solution (pH5), and ninhydrin reagent. The mixture is refluxed in a water bath for thirty minutes, cooled to 21.8 $^\circ$C, and diluted with isopropanol to a total volume of 10ml. Light absorbance readings are determined using a spectrometer.

Advantages:

- The Ninhydrin colorimetric reaction is a simple, rapid, and inexpensive method.

Salivary amine levels measured by the Ninhydrin method significantly correlated with organoleptic scores and sulphide monitor measurements in halitosis patients and control subjects.

10) Polymerase chain reaction

Real-time polymerase chain reaction (PCR) using the TaqMan system can be used for quantitative analysis of volatile sulphur-containing compounds producing oral bacteria.

An oligonucleotide probe with a reporter fluorescent dye attached to its 50-end and a quencher dye attached to its 30-end is designed to hybridize to the target gene. During PCR amplification, the quencher dye of the probe is cleaved by the 50- nuclease activity of Taq polymerase, resulting in the accumulation of reporter fluorescence. The release of the fluorescent dye during amplification allows for the rapid detection and quantification of oral bacteria DNA.[3]

Using the polymerase chain reaction, a strong correlation was found between the presence of *Bacteroides forsythus* in saliva of subjects with periodontitis and the concentration of volatile sulphur-containing compounds in breath air measured using gas chromatography.

11) Tongue Sulfide Probe

Sensors for volatile sulfur compounds have been integrated into periodontal probes and paddles which can be placed directly into the pocket or onto the tongue, again yielding significant co-relation with organoleptic scores. The tongue sulfide probe size is 0.25 x 0.75 inches and was developed to determine the sulfide levels on the tongue dorsum (pS level). It is composed of an active sulfide sensing element and a stable sulfide element.

Method:

The tongue sulfide probe is applied on the anterior, middle or the posterior part of the tongue along the median groove of the tongue dorsum with a light pressure for 30sec. The sulfide-sensing element generates an electrochemical voltage proportional to the concentration of sulfide ions present. The voltage is measured relative to the operating point of reference element. The electrochemical voltage generated by the sulfide is measured by the electronic unit, and are displayed in a digital score ranging from 0.0 (undetectable pS: less than 10^{-7} M of sulfide) to 0.5 (more than equal to 10^{-2} M of sulfide) in increments of 0.5.

It has been shown that the tongue sulfide levels assessed with this probe were significantly co-related with whole mouth odor. It appears to be a simple, reliable and clinically user friendly tool for assessing oral malodor, more specifically.[70]

12) Zinc Oxide Thin Film Conductor Sensor

This device, which is used to diagnose oral malodor in clinics, was devised by Shimura and Company in 1996. The results obtained by this device co-related with the values of total volatile sulfur compounds measured by Gas Chromatography and also with organoleptic scores given by the judges.

The apparatus casing is Zinc oxide thin film semiconductor sensor. The system is composed of a gas intake part. Sensor detector, control panel and digital display of the output.The gas intake part is walled within Teflon material and tubing that absorbs the least amount of organic matter. Sample gas is taken up by a motorized pump through the Teflon inlet and is altered by a rinsing cycle activated by an electromagnetic valve. A special acidic silica gel filter that traps ketones and alcohols is inserted in the inlet part. Each step operation and the lapse time are indicated by the digital display on control panel. The output is also numerically expressed on the panel. [71]

Advantages:

- Small size
- Simple to handle
- Responds specifically to several volatile sulfur
- compounds in mouth air.
- Highly sensitive

- Can measure halitosis due to non-volatile sulfur compounds
- Could be used for diagnosis of diabetes as it measures acetone in mouth air.

Disadvantage:

- It does not discriminate between gases, but presents the measures as a total gas mixture hence exaggerated readings are obtained.

13) Ora Test (Figure XIV)

This test was developed by **Rosenberg et al.**[72] it provides quantitative assessment of the level of microbial activity in the oral cavity. The test involves oral rinsing with a sterile milk sample, followed by expectoration into a test tube containing a oxidation-reduction reduction indicator (methyleneblue). The higher level of micro-organisms, the faster the color changes from blue (aerobic condition) to white anaerobic condition at the bottom of the test tube. In addition to co-relation with microbial counts, the OraTest exhibits significant co-relation with plaque and gingival indices.

Figure XIV: Ora Test

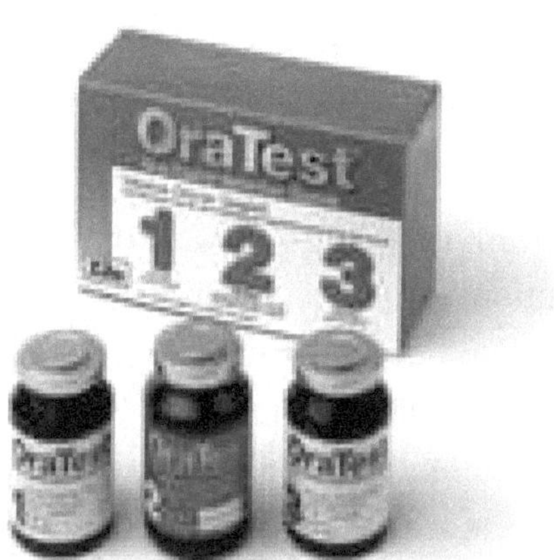

14) Self-assessment of oral malodor

The age-old method of breathing into the cupped palms to discern one's own breath may or may not detect anything. Regardless, if foulness is detected by this antiquated method, rating its severity and improvement/degradation over time is not possible in this way. The value in self-diagnosing may be in establishing a suspicion of a problem.

Methods:

A) By licking the wrist with the length of the tongue (including as far back as possible) and waiting 5 seconds before sniff-testing, one is allegedly able to discern negligible or problematic tongue odors.

B) By doing the same with floss, one can detect

negligible or problematic periodontal odors.

C) By having another person evaluate mouth breath (while nose pinched closed) versus nose expirations (while holding mouth closed) can help detect odors of sinus origin.

D) OK-to-Kiss (Emjoi)[6] was a palate and treatment solution kit. It had a novel color change that correlated to an enzyme that related to one's malodor status. The kit is no longer marketed because of its high price.

E) Subjects are asked to score their own oral malodor on a continuous 10cm visual analogue scale (VAS) marked on each end as "no odor" and "extremely foul odor", respectively. Five self-assessments were made:

(i) *Preconception score-* prior to measurement, subjects asked to score the level of bad breath which they thought they had at that time.

(ii) *Whole-mouth malodor score-* subjects are instructed to smell the odor emanating from their entire mouth by cupping their hands over mouth and nose, exhaling through the mouth, and breathing in through the nose;

(iii) *Tongue malodor score-* subjects are asked to extend their tongue and lick their wrist in a perpendicular fashion (Odor was judged by smelling the wrist after 5 sec at a distance of 3 cm)

(iv) *Saliva malodor score-* saliva samples (1ml), obtained by expectoration is allowed to stand in closed Petri dishes for 5 min at 37°C and then presented for odor assessment at a distance of 4 cm.

(v) *Post measurement score-* Immediately following the various self-assessments, subjects are again asked to rate their own oral malodor. In each instance, subjects are blinded to all previous scores. Finally, as a control to assess the subjects' scoring of a given foul odor, chicken-dung-based fertilizer (Kuftigal, Haifa, Israel) in aqueous suspension is presented to the subjects and the odor judge in an opaque sniff bottle and scored on the 10cm visual analogue scale.[73]

TREATMENT

Successful treatment of halitosis depends on a correct diagnosis and the implementation of a cause related therapy.[83] The first step in treating oral malodor is to assess all oral diseases and conditions that may contribute to oral malodor. For disease-free people, oral malodor treatment is based on the assumption that the malodor is the result of an overgrowth of oral microorganisms, which produce volatile compounds that are offensive. The aim of the treatment is to reduce these microorganisms in the oral cavity, with concomitant reduction in the formation of volatile compounds. This may be accomplished by mechanical or chemical methods.[10]

The simplest way to distinguish oral from non-oral etiologies is to compare the smell coming from the patient's mouth with that exiting the nose. If the odor is primarily from the mouth, an oral origin may be inferred.[6]

TREATMENT NEEDS

CLASSIFICATION OF HALITOSIS WITH CORRESPONDING TREATMENT NEEDS (TN)

Classification	**Treatment Needs (TN)**
1. Genuine halitosis	
a. Physiologic Halitosis	TN-1 b. Pathologic Halitosis
(i) Oral	TN-1, 2
(ii) Extraoral	TN-1, 3
2. Pseudo Halitosis	TN-1, 4
3. Halitophobia	TN-1, 5

Treatment needs (TN) for breath malodor

TN-1: Explanation of halitosis and instructions for oral hygiene (support and reinforcement of a patient's own self-care for further improvement of their oral hygiene).

TN-2: Oral prophylaxis, professional cleaning and treatment for oral diseases, especially periodontal diseases.

TN-3: Referral to a physician or medical specialist.

TN-4: Explanation of examination data, further professional instruction, education and reassurance.

TN-5: Referral to a clinical psychologist, psychiatrist or other psychological specialist.

Treatment Needs-1 (TN-1)

Physiological halitosis mainly originates from the dorsoposterior region of the tongue, and the malodor is derived from the tongue coating. Therefore, in TN-1, cleaning the tongue is more important than rinsing the mouth. The tongue coating comprises of desquamated epithelial cells, blood cells and bacteria. More than 100 bacteria may be attached to a single epithelial cell on the tongue dorsum, where as only about 25 bacteria are attached to eachcell in other areas of the oral cavity. Hence, cleaning the tongue is a very effective measure for improving physiologic halitosis. It has been reported by that mechanical stimulation enhances carcinogenesis of the tongue in experimental animals.[34] Patients with psychological conditions may overzealously scrape or brush the tongue till bleeding starts; therefore, detailed, comprehensive instruction about tongue cleaning should be given. The position of the terminal sulcus of the tongue and the anatomical limits for cleaning should be known and demonstrated so as to not to brush or scrape the tongue tonsil. The remaining treatments in TN-1 include routine oral hygiene procedures and mouth rinsing. Research articles on North American mouthwashes containing zinc, chlorhexidine and hydrogen peroxide indicate the efficacy of these agents in reducing malodour. The side effects of chlorhexidine mouthwash include tooth stains and allergic reaction, and the oxidative activity of hydrogen peroxide might be harmful to the oral soft tissues. Therefore, it is recommended to use a mouthwash containing zinc.[34]

Morning bad breath in healthy subjects is a cosmetic problem analogous to body malodor. Morning bad breath develops during sleep when the saliva flow rate and the oxygen availability are at their lowest, promoting anaerobic formation of Volatile Sulfur Compounds. To reduce morning bad breath tongue scraping is advised in the evening before sleeping.

Mouthrinses are also advocated to reduce morning bad breath. After drinking and eating in the morning the halitosis will most likely disappear.[2]

Treatment Needs-2 (TN-2)

Oral pathologic halitosis is caused mainly by periodontal disease, a condition managed by periodontal treatment. Additionally, dental treatment may be necessary to correct faulty restorations that might contribute to poor oral health.[34]

Treatment Needs-3 (TN-3)

Patients exhibiting oral malodour but showing no oral cause of halitosis are classified as having extraoral pathologic halitosis, and they should be referred to medical specialists.[34] Therapy for Trimethylaminuria is limited. It appears that dietary management might be most effective in mild to moderate forms of fish odor syndrome but not in all cases. Halitosis associated with medication need to be discussed with the patient's physician.[2]

Treatment Needs-4 (TN-4)

Patients with pseudo-halitosis mistakenly believe that

other individuals' avoidance behaviors are caused by their own oral malodour. Hence, counseling, with literature support, education and explanation of examination results that the intensity of their malodor is not beyond a socially acceptable level is to be done. This step is most important in differentiating pseudo-halitosis from Halitophobia. Pseudo-halitosis patients generally respond favorably to TN-4 because they can accept the counselling.[34] The therapeutic recommendation is never to advise to use certain products against halitosis. Patients with the experience of tonsilloliths also can develop a Halitophobia.[2]

Treatment Needs-5 (TN-5)

Patients who cannot accept their perception of malodor as a mistaken belief are classified as halitophobic and need assistance from a psychological specialist (TN-5). Furthermore, patients with genuine halitosis who undergo successful reduction of halitosis by TN-2 or TN-3 yet still believe that they have the condition should also be referred to a psychological specialist. Halitophobic patients usually refuse to visit a psychological specialist, because they cannot recognize their condition as psychosomatic. It is important, therefore, to provide TN-4 counseling to halitophobic patients.[34]

TREATMENT APPROACHES FOR ORAL MALODOR

A. Mechanical Approach
B. Chemical Approach
C. Conversion of Volatile Sulfur Compounds
D. Masking the Malodor
E. Lethal photosensitization
F. Probiotics

A. MECHANICAL APPROACH

1. Tongue Scraping (Figure XV)

The importance of mechanical tongue cleaning as an oral hygiene procedure has gained new interest because it has been shown that bacterial tongue coating is an important source for Volatile Sulfur Compound, which are major components in oral malodor.[84] Several studies[6,83,85] have implicated the dorsum of the tongue as the primary source of Volatile Sulfur Compound, both in periodontally diseased and healthy individual. Researchers have been able to find positive correlations between tongue coating status (amount and or presence) and the different parameters directly related with oral malodor.[84] Thus tongue becomes the most important micro environment to study and to target in the prevention and treatment of oral halitosis and also as a potential reservoir for periodontal pathogens.

A fissured tongue is associated with oral malodor, presumably because it provides an increased surface area for bacteria to colonize. But it could also provide an increased surface for leakage of host molecules into the saliva. This suggests that the tongue surface itself may be the main source of nutrients for the bacteria in the tongue coating, and that a vicious cycle of bacterial growth leading to host inflammation, resulting into bacterial overgrowth further leading to more inflammation. This cycle can be interrupted by careful debridement of the tongue either by brushing or by using a plastic device to gently scrape the coating from the posterior of the tongue.[30]

Numerous studies[30,34] have found a relationship between the mechanical removal of tongue coating and the reduction of both organoleptic scores and Volatile Sulfur Compound levels, including reduction in methyl mercaptan levels and the methyl mercaptan/hydrogen sulfide ratio, in both healthy and periodontitis patients, with or without halitosis. Mechanical reduction of malodor and of the intraoral bacterial count may be achieved by disrupting the tongue biofilm, thus decreasing the production of Volatile Sulfur Compounds and other volatile organic compounds.

Various available instruments can be applied to the tongue, and by gentle pressure the majority of the tongue coating can be scraped off. Brushing the dorsum of the tongue with toothpaste is more effective than brushing the teeth. The duration of these effects varies from 15 to 100 minutes and depends on the device used to remove the coating, i.e., toothbrush or *tonguescraper*, lasting longer for tongue scrapers than for toothbrushes.[40]

Scraping is a very important action in removing debris from the tongue; brushing also maybe important as a pre-cleaning procedure that loosens debris in deeper areas of the tongue. Therefore, a combination of brushing five times and scraping five times with a tongue cleaner may be slightly more effective than performing either procedure 10 times.[84] Single scraping of the tongue with a plastic strip have minimal impact on tongue streptococcal numbers.[86]

Figure XV: One Drop Only Tongue Cleaner (One Drop Only GmbH, Berlin) (a combination brush and scraper)

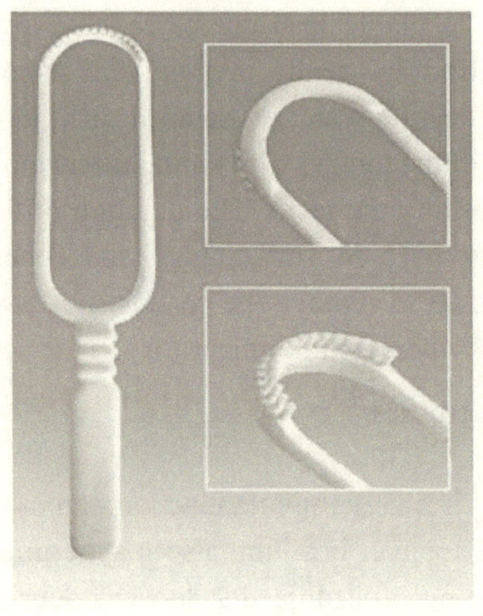

The percentage of Volatile Sulfur Compound reduction has been related to the different devices used, ranging from 33% with a toothbrush, to 42% with a specially designed tongue cleaner; and also to the periodontal health status, being higher for halitosis patients without periodontal disease (51.8%) than for periodontitis patients (49%).

A study by Seeman R et al.[84] found a relationship

between tongue cleaning and the reduction of both organoleptic scores and levels of volatile sulphur-containing compounds. In patients with high levels of oral malodor, a regular toothbrush was statistically significantly less effective in tongue cleaning than a device that brushed and scraped, orascraper. Because of the limited duration of the effect, efficacy remained questionable.

Two weeks of tongue brushing or scraping by a group of patients free of periodontitis resulted in negligible reductions in bacteria on the tongue, whereas the amount of tongue coating decreased significantly. Therefore, tongue cleaning seems to reduce the substrates for putrefaction, rather than the bacterial load.[40]

According to Cochrane Database of Systematic Reviews[87] there is weak and unreliable evidence to show that there is a small but statistically significant difference in reduction of Volatile Sulfur Compound levels when tongue scrapers or cleaners rather than tooth brushes are used to reduce halitosis in adults.

And no high level evidence was found comparing mechanical with other forms of tongue cleaning.

2. Tooth Brushing and Interdental Cleaning

Mechanical cleaning of teeth, such as brushing the teeth and flossing reduced the amount of oral bacteria and substrates, thereby presumably reducing oral malodor. Interdental cleaning and tooth brushing removes residual food particles and organisms that cause putrefaction. It has been stated that using a regular toothbrush for tongue cleaning is inferior for removing debris and organisms from the tongue compared with using a scraping debridement tool and it is desirable to use a product that provides maximum effect with a minimum number of movements on the tongue, thus reducing the gagging reflex.[84]

In subjects free of caries, periodontal disease and tongue coating, brushing the teeth exclusively had no appreciable influence on the concentration of volatile sulfur containing compounds in morning breath, when compared with no brushing and rinsing the mouth with water. Since periodontitis can be a factor in chronic oral malodor, professional periodontal treatment is mandatory. Thus, initial periodontal therapy in moderate periodontitis patients can be expected to improve breath odor parameters by reducing the number of period on to pathogens.[53,88]

However, it has been proposed that interdental flossing has no added value with regard to reducing morning bad breath.[40] Clinical studies revealed that brushing the teeth exclusively was not very effective in reducing oral malodor scores. A combination of tooth and tongue brushing or tooth brushing alone have a beneficial effect on bad breath for up to 1 hour (73% and 30% reductions in VSC, respectively).

B. CHEMICAL APPROACH

The goal of any antimicrobial treatment would be to reduce the proteolytic, anaerobic flora found on the tongue surface.[40]

Mouth rinses with antimicrobial properties can reduce oral malodor by reducing the number of microorganisms chemically. Often used active ingredients in these products are chlorhexidine (CHX), essential oils (EOs), and triclosan and cetylpyridinium chloride (CPC). Mouth rinses can also reduce halitosis by chemically neutralizing odorcompounds, including Volatile Sulfur Compounds. Often used active ingredients of these Products are metal ions and oxidizing agents.[40]

1. Chlorhexidine (Figure XVI)

Chlorhexidine gluconate is a cationic bis-biguanide, with a broad antimicrobial spectrum and has been approved by the American Dental Association. Results from a case series study by **DeBoever EH et al.**[47] in halitosis patients suggested a significant effect of Chlorhexidine rinsing and tongue brushing on halitosis reduction after1 week of treatment. In studies by **van Stenberghe et al.**[89] **and Carvalho MD et al.**[90] 0.2% Chlorhexidine mouth rinse produced significant reductions in volatile sulfur- containing compound levels and organoleptic scores. Similar results with 0.12% Chlorhexidine-(di) gluconate are reported by **DeBoever EH et al.**[47] in combination with teeth and tongue brushing. Due to its substantivity, the anti-Volatile Sulfur Compound effect of the 0.2% solution is satisfactory after 1 hour but, more importantly, it shows a tendency to improve at 2 hour and 3 hour. A commercial product containing0.12% Chlorhexidine-gluconate is demonstrated as an effective anti-Volatile Sulfur Compound product, and shows kinetics similar to that of the 0.2% Chlorhexidine solution. Although Chlorhexidine is considered the gold standard mouthrinse for halitosis treatment, it has undesirable side effects. According to a study by **Bosy A et al.**[91] ninety of one hundred and one patients who used the 0.2% Chlorhexidine rinse for 1 week responded to a questionnaire concerning adverse reactions. Eighty-eight percent of the patients had at least one complaint, with 59% experiencing a change in the taste of food and 25% experiencing a burning sensation at the tip of the tongue. About 4% of the subjects reported sloughing of the tissues or gingival pain, which would be a more serious concern. An agent is needed that approaches the clinical efficacy of Chlorhexidine but with better safety and comfort features.

Figure XVI: PerioGard 0.12% Chlorhexidine Mouthrinse (Colgate Pharmaceuticals)™

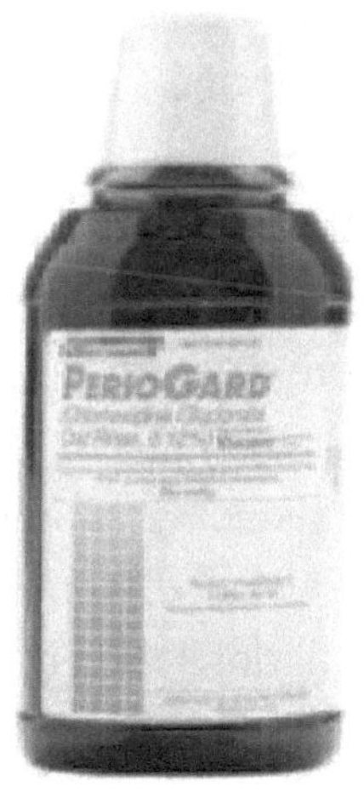

2. Essential oils (Figure XVII)

Essential oils (EO), including hydro-alcohol solutions of thymol, menthol, eucalyptol, and methyl salicylate, are used in mouthwashes to prevent periodontal disease. Their anti-plaque and anti-gingivitis activity is well known. Re-odoration is important to the overall activity of the product only for about 30 min after treatment and, at post-treatment times of 60-180 min, the anti-odor activity of the product is due to its anti-microbial action. This is the basis for the premise that anti-Volatile Sulfur Compound agents would succeed if they had an anti microbial component.[92] Rinsing with an Essential oils mouth rinse can have long lasting effects in reducing anaerobic bacteria overall as well as Gram-negative anaerobes and Volatile Sulfur Compound producing bacteria. The significant reductions in numbers of these bacteria produced by the Essential oil mouth rinse, both in plaque and on the dorsum of the tongue, can play a key role in explaining the Essential oil mouth rinse's effectiveness in reducing supragingival plaque and gingivitis as well as its effectiveness in controlling intrinsic oral malodor. According to a study conducted by **Pitts G et al.**[92] an Essential oil mouth rinse is able to reduce the offensive gases present in morning bad breath as measured by a reduction of the organoleptic scores, and caused a sustained reduction in the plaque odorigenic bacteria.

Figure XVII: Thieves Fresh Essence Plus Essential Oils Mouthwash (Young Living)^{TM}

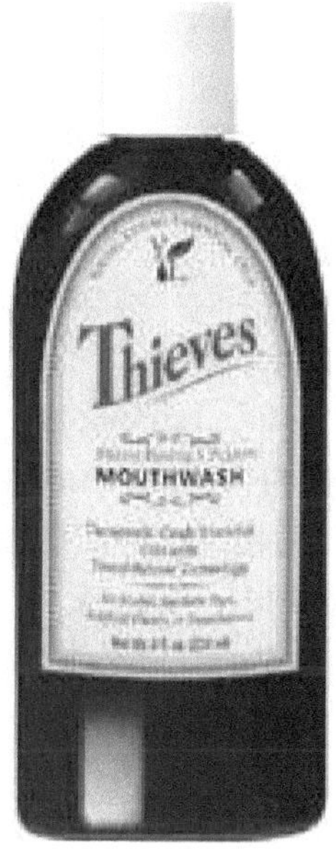

3. Triclosan (Figure XVIII)

The clinical experiments performed by Young et al.[93] showed that mouth-rinsing with triclosan solubilized in sodium lauryl sulfate, propylene glycol and water gave a marked and long-lasting anti-Volatile Sulfur Compound effect. The in vitro experiment supported the contention that triclosan exhibitsan anti-Volatile Sulfur Compound effect per se. Carvalho et al.[90] reported that triclosan and Cetylpyridinium mouth rinses were more effective in reducing bad breath than in reducing supragingival plaque accumulation. Therefore, it is postulated that the superior reducing effect of these specific mouth rinses on bad breath may be related primarily to their efficacy in reducing the load of Volatile Sulfur Compound-related microorganisms and oral debris in the whole mouth niches rather than only in supragingival plaque reduction.

Figure XVIII: Minty Citrus Splash (Cetylpyridinium Chloride and Triclosan) Mouthwash (Dentyl pH)^{TM}

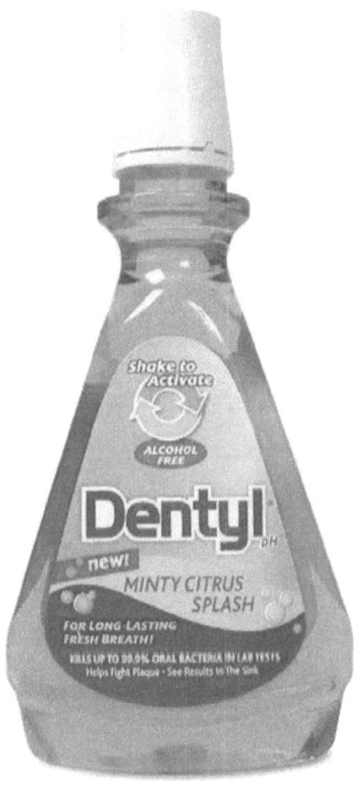

4. Cetyl pyridinium chloride (Figure XIX)

Quaternary ammonium compounds, such as benzalkonium and cetylpyridinium chloride, inhibit bacterial growth, but the results are modest for plaque and equivocal for gingivitis. A Cetylpyridinium chloride (CPC) rinse used in a 6-week pre-brushing study by Moran J et al.[94] failed to confer any adjunctive benefit to oral hygiene and gingival health compared to a control rinse. Debate is still going over the action of cationic antiseptics in the oral cavity. Studies by Caravalho MD et al.[90] and Young A et al.[95] also demonstrated that the Cetylpyridinium mouthrinse presents the lowest impact in reducing Volatile Sulfur Compounds of morning breath when compared with other products and is supported by the observation that this quaternary ammonium compound agent is not substantive enough to promote an essential antibacterial activity. Substantivity of Cetylpyridinium is 3 hours, therefore, a frequent use of Cetyl pyridinium could improve plaque inhibition but it can lead to compliance problems.

Figure XIX: Vitis (Cetylpyridinium Chloride) Mouthwash (Vitis)^{TM}

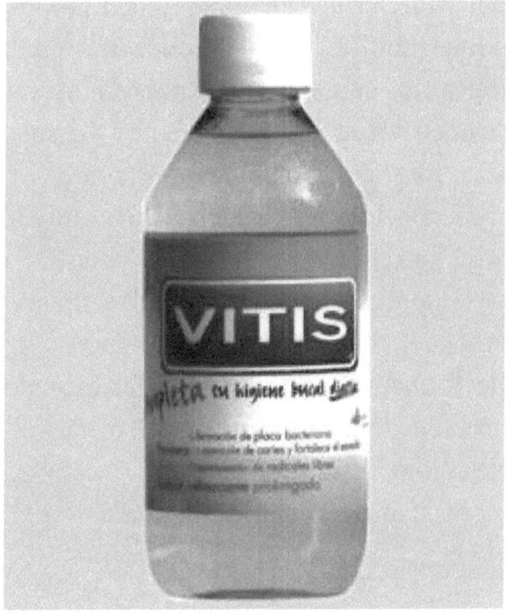

5. Zinc (Figure XX)

Metals such as zinc, sodium, tin and magnesium interact with sulfur. The mechanism proposed is that metal ions oxidize the thiol groups in the precursors of volatile sulfur containing compounds. Morning breath odor can be successfully reduced by the sole use of an amine fluoride stannous fluoride containing mouthrinse twice daily, which significantly reduces the bacterial load in the saliva and retards the denovo plaque formation. Both cupric and stannous ions have the potential to discolor teeth, either as a result of sulfide formation on the teeth after extended periods of use or due to the precipitation of dietary chromogen. Cupric chloride is the most effective metal solution for inhibiting hydrogen sulfide production at 1, 2 and 3 hours after rinsing.[40]

Zinc is the metal ion of choice with this purpose because of its low toxicity and its other favorable properties, such as not causing dental staining. Zinc ions possessing anti- Volatile Sulfur Compound effects have affinity for sulfur, forming sulfides with low solubility. Oral products containing zinc are also effective in reducing or inhibiting oral malodor. In a study conducted by Young et al.[95] 1% zinc acetate solution had excellent anti-Volatile Sulfur Compound effect throughout the test period of 3 hour, although the metallic taste experienced at this concentration was a little unpleasant. This problem is overcome in commercial products by masking it with other ingredients.

Figure XX: Smart Mouth (Zinc Mouthwash) Smart Mouth^{TM}

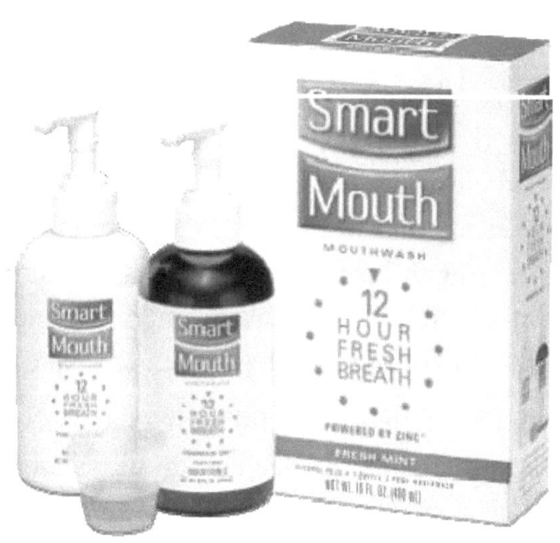

6. Chlorine Dioxide (Figure XXI)

Chlorine dioxide, a strong oxidizing agent, consumes oral substrates containing cysteine and methionine, thus preventing the production of Volatile Sulfur Compounds. A study by Frascella J et al.[96] evaluated the effect of a commercially available chlorine dioxide mouthrinse on Volatile Sulfur Compounds levels in a panel of healthy subjects. The results of the investigation demonstrated a beneficial effect of a chlorine dioxide mouthrinse on Volatile Sulfur Compound control in the morning breath of healthy subjects. The subjects of the study conducted by Richter JL[97] were instructed as to how to floss their teeth, to clean the posterior third of the tongue with a tongue blade and to rinse with a proprietary chlorine dioxide mouthrinse. Seventy eight percent of the individuals felt a significant improvement in their breath odor problem. A higher success rate has been reported by Richter JL[97] following the use of an intra oral liquid-airspray device and an ultrasonic intraoral dental cleaner modified to deliver a 20 ppm molecular chlorine dioxide irrigant to the hard and soft tissues of the mouth.

Figure XXI: CloSYS (Chlorine Dioxide) Antiseptic Oral Rinse (Rowpar Pharmaceuticals)[TM]

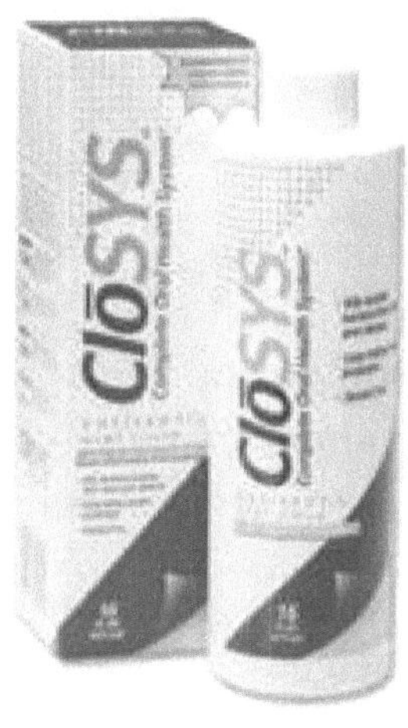

Effective Combination of agents

7. Chlorhexidine and zinc

A Chlorhexidine and zinc mouthrinse has a strong effect on volatile sulfur-containing compounds and is effective for at least 9 hours. Control rinses with Chlorhexidine or zinc alone have a moderate and strong effect for 1 hour, but this effect diminishes with time.[95]

8. Cetylpyridinium and zinc ions

A Cetylpyridinium and zinc mouthrinse have a good synergistic effect on volatile sulfur-containing compounds levels after 1 hour, but minimally above the effect of zinc alone.[95]

9. Chlorhexidine, cetylpyridinium chloride and zinc-lactate

Chlorhexidine is considered the gold standard mouthrinse, but it does have some side effects. Due to these disadvantages, new formulations have been developed. Since Chlorhexidine and Cetylpyridinium are both antimicrobial agents, it seems reasonable to assume a mouthwash that contains Chlorhexidine and Cetylpyridinium acts by reducing the number of Volatile Sulfur Compound -producing bacteria on the dorsum of the tongue. Moreover, zinc-lactate, besides its antimicrobial activity, may reduce Volatile Sulfur Compound scores by transforming them into insoluble compounds. Two dual-centers, double-blind, placebo-controlled studies conducted by Roldan S et al.[85,98] demonstrated that a mouthwash containing Chlorhexidine(0.05%), Cetylpyridinium(0.05%) and zinc-lactate(0.14%) is effective in the treatment of oral halitosis. The one adverse effect of the active mouthwash was staining of the dorsum of the tongue.

It has been indicated that there is a synergistic action between Chlorhexidine and cetylpyridine. The replacement of alcohol in a Chlorhexidine formulation by Cetylpyridinium does not change the antimicrobial activity of the mouthrinse, even though the Chlorhexidine concentration is reduced to 0.05%. A 0.12% Chlorhexidine and 0.05% cetylpyridinium solution was compared by Roldan S et al.[99] to a 0.05% Chlorhexidine, 0.05% Cetylpyridinium and 0.14% zinc-lactate solution, and to other 3 different commercial mouthrinses with Chlorhexidine. Formulations combining Chlorhexidine and Cetylpyridinium achieved the best results, both in terms of anti-microbial activity and anti-halitosis efficacy. Conversely, a formulation combining Chlorhexidine with sodium flouride showed significantly lower anti-halitosis and anti-microbial efficacy.

C. CONVERSION OF VOLATILE SULFUR COMPOUNDS

1. Metal Salt Solutions

Metal ions with affinity for sulfur are rather efficient in capturing the sulfur containing gases. Zinc is an ion with two positive charges, which will bind to the twice-negatively loaded sulfur radicles, and thus can reduce the expression of the Volatile Sulfur Compounds. The same applies for other metalions, such as mercury and copper. Clinically, the inhibitory effect is *copper dichloride> stannous fluoride> zinc dichloride*. In vitro, the inhibitory effect was *mercury dichloride=copper dichloride =cadmium chloride> zinc dichloride> stannous fluoride> stannous dichloride> lead dichloride*. *Halita*, mouth rinse containing 0.05% Chlorhexidine, 0.05% Cetylpyridinium, and 0.14% zinc lactate, has been even more efficient than a 0.2% Chlorhexidine formulation in reducing the Volatile Sulfur Compound levels and organoleptic ratings. The special effect of Halita may result from the Volatile Sulfur Compound conversion ability of zinc, besides its antimicrobial action.[7]

2. Toothpastes

Baking soda dentifrices have been shown to be effective with a 44% reduction of Volatile Sulfur Compound levels 3 hours after tooth brushing versus a 31% reduction of a fluoride dentifrice. The mechanism by which baking soda produces its inhibition of oral malodor might be related to its bactericidal effects and its transformation of Volatile Sulfur Compounds to a nonvolatile state.[7]

3. Chewing Gum (Figure XXII)

Chewing gum can be formulated with antibacterial agents, such as fluoride or chlorhexidine, thus helping in reducing oral malodor through both mechanical and chemical approaches. A beneficial effect of chewing gum containing tea extracts for its deodorizing mechanism has been investigated and Epigallocatchin (EGCg) has been reported as the main deodorizing agent among the tea catechins. The chemical reaction between Epigallocatchin and Methyl Mercaptan results in non- volatile product.[7]

Figure XXII: Mega-T Green Tea Chewing Gum
(CCA Pharmaceuticals)

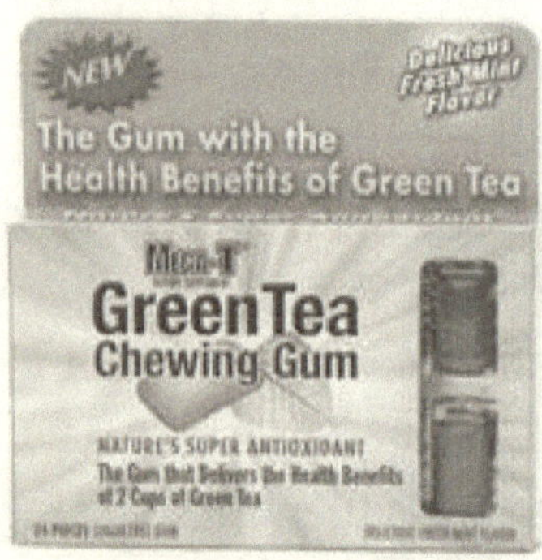

D. MASKING THE MALODOR

Treatments with rinses, mouth sprays, and lozenges containing volatiles with a pleasant odor have only a short term effect for example mint containing lozenges. Another pathway is to increase the solubility of malodorous compounds in the saliva by lowering the pH of the saliva (low pH increases the solubility of Volatile Sulfur Compounds) or simply increase the secretion of saliva; a larger volume allows the retention of larger volumes of soluble Volatile Sulfur Compounds. The latter can also be achieved by ensuring a proper liquid intake or by using a chewing gum; chewing triggers the periodontal-parotid reflex, atleast when the lower premolars are still present. To lower the pH, an orange juice may be sufficient, but the effect is short term.

E. LETHAL PHOTOSENSITIZATION

Photodynamic therapy is a relatively new treatment modality, which was primarily used to destroy tumor cells with the power of laser light energy. Targeting the power to the pathologic cells was reached by staining them with specific dyes that are able to selectively absorb light energy of certain wavelength and are accumulated by tumor cells in lager quantities than by normal cells. The same principle, named lethal photosensitization, using different dyes (photosensitizer) was later applied to killing different species of bacteria witha significant level of success.

Lethal photosensitization is a process by which a photosensitizer is activated by light of an appropriate wavelength resulting in the production of cytotoxic oxygen free radical species, which then kill the target cell. Lethal photosensitization is not a specific modality and has been shown to be effective against a variety of cells such as those in neoplasms, fungi, viruses, and bacteria. Bacteria are killed as a result of membrane and DNA damage due mainly to the production of singlet oxygen on irradiation of the dye.[9]

Development of resistance to photodynamic therapy would appear to be unlikely since its bactericidal activity is due to single oxygen and other reactive species such as hydroxyl radicals, which affect a range of cellular targets. Lethal photosensitization is not specific is advantageous in one respect; it is possible to kill all the bacteria present in a mixed infection. However, this also means that commensal bacteria and host tissues could be adversely affected, especially with high-density local power output of the laser light sources.

KrespiYP et al.[9] in a study on Lethal Photosensitization of two common oral pathogens *Porphyromonas gingivalis* and *Prevotella intermedia* viared-filtered halogen lamp found that exposure of these bacterial cultures to red-filtered high-intensity light for less than 10 min in combination with exposure to Methylene Blue solution at a concentration of 0.01% and higher, produced significant bactericidal effect on both species. They also found that exposure to red light with wavelength of 650 nm alone does not produce any significant killing in *Prevotella intermedia* and *Porphyromonas gingivalis*.

F. PROBIOTICS (Figure XXIII)

Probiotics, defined by the World Health Organization as 'live microorganisms which when administered in adequate amounts confer a health benefit on the host', may provide a supplementary treatment. Antimicrobial treatment indiscriminately depletes populations of both the problematic bacteria and those bacteria that are not thought to be implicated in halitosis, but which are likely to be important in the maintenance of a normal oral micro environment. Given that the dorsum of the tongue is the origin of most malodor problems, a candidate probiotic to counter this condition should be able to persist within this particular ecosystem.

Streptococcus salivarius strains appear to be excellent candidates for an oral probiotic, since they are early colonizers of oral surfaces and are amongst the most numerically-predominant members of the tongue microbiota of 'healthy' individuals. This species also has only a limited ability to produce volatile sulphur compounds and is unlikely to contribute significantly to oral odour. *Streptococcus salivarius* has not been implicated either in caries or in other infectious diseases of humans. Characteristics of *S.salivarius* strains for their potential application as oral probiotics includes: bacteriocins, persistence in the oral cavity, adhesion to various oral cells and viability on freeze drying and storage. *Streptococcus salivarius* strain K12 is considered to be a particularly good candidate, since it produces at least two 1 antibiotic-type bacteriocins which are especially potent against gram-positive bacteria.

A series of bacterial strains representative of species implicated in halitosis were tested by Burton et al. to see if they were inhibited by the two bacteriocins produced by strain K12. Inhibition was observed for *Streptococcus anginosis*, *Eubacterium saburreum* and *Micromonas micros*, but not for *Porphyromonas gingivalis* and *Prevotella intermedia*. But when fresh saliva was inoculated onto agar medium impregnated with the bacteriocins produced by strain K12, inhibition of black-pigmented bacteria identified as *Prevotella species* was observed. In a Pilot Study by Burton et al.[100] a course of lozenges containing strain K12 were taken by 13 subjects with confirmed halitosis following mouth-rinsing with chlorhexidine. When measured after 1 week of using the K12 lozenges (4 days after ceasing use of the chlorhexidine), 11 of the subjects had volatile sulphur readings that were reduced by atleast 100 ppb when compared with pretreatment levels. Eight subjects maintained substantially reduced Volatile Sulfur Compound levels for at least 14 days. All subjects showed an increase in the levels of *Streptococcus salivarius* as a proportion of their total salivary populations and other measures of halitosis such as BANA reactivity and organoleptic scores were reduced. But the mechanism(s) of volatile sulphur compound reduction could not be clearly established.

FIGURE XXII: Aktiv-K12 Probiotic

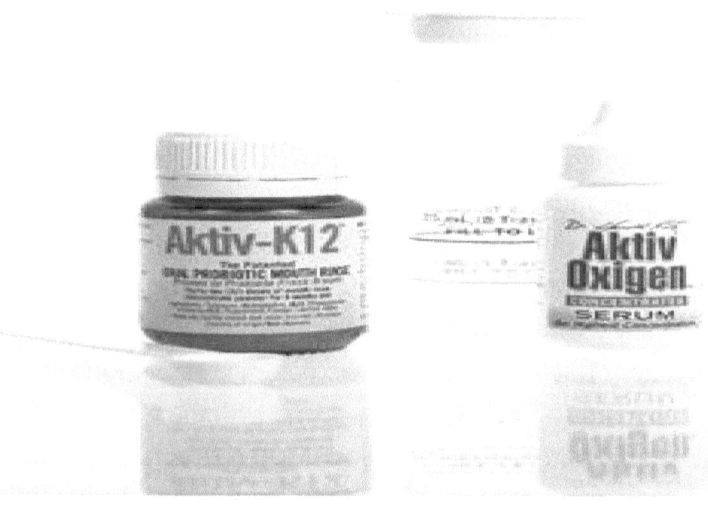

PUBLIC HEALTH SIGNIFICANCE OF HALITOSIS

In the society, there is constant pressure to look and smell good; halitosis is undesirable. It is a crippling social problem with a common complaint of up to one-third of the general population. Today it is widely recognized that the sense of smell is closely linked to our memory and basic emotions. Perception of odors in human olfactory system is thus important in the creation and conservation of social bonds, as they are loaded with cultural values.[85]

The olfactory, smelling experience is emotionally charged and helps to connects us with the world.[86] The smell from mouth, breath odor can consequently either connect or disconnect a person from his or her social environment and social relationships. Halitosis is one of society's oldest and most troublesome social maladies. It is a common and universal affliction suffered by many people irrespective of age, sex, social status. Over half of the population experiences it but only one out of ten adults suffers from its severity that requires medical help.[1]

Halitosis has become a major health concern among the general public because it causes significant amount of social disharmony, embarrassment, frustration, despair and often leads toward social and professional isolation and marital problems.[84] Bad breath is known to have a devastating effect on the daily social life of those who suffer from it[87] thus earning the title 'social life killer'. In western societies, embarrassment and discomfort are the main reasons for seeking professional care. Because society quickly develops a negative towards those with halitosis, it can be a very influential factor in a person's life.

Halitosis may be an important factor in social communication hence the origin of concern is not only due to a possible health condition, but also psychological alterations leading to social and personal isolation.

The psychological and social impacts of genuine and delusional halitosis are mentioned as under:[88]

Bad Breath and Relationships-
Bad breath and relationships are similar to oil and water: they don't mix. Halitosis can put a severe strain on all types of relationships, be it social, personal or intimate. And bad breath can be a key factor when beginning a new relationship or keeping one going. Broaching the subject of bad breath, even with a partner, can be extremely difficult and is often avoided until the problem reaches a point where it can no longer be overlooked.[1] Bad breath is a huge social issue; it causes embarrassment and creates a social barrier between themselves and their loved ones,

relatives, friends and colleagues. Friend circle or peer group is most venerable social group for any person and highly important for young adults mainly 2 type of response can be expected-
1. Positive feedback response
2. Negative feedback response.
In positive feedback response, a friend can give a good advice such as a visit a doctors but in negative feedback response are generally very harmful for the affected person here, they make jokes on the person without understanding the problem or without thinking that how the affected person will react to this usually peer group comments are very sensitive for all of us so affected person could be pushed into depression sometimes, leading to fatal outcome.

Possible psychological outcomes of chronic malodor maybe:[84]
Socially Isolation- Affected person may get depressed by others comments and makes psychological barriers, making him/herself socially isolated so that he/she get less chance to interact with others, avoiding social embarrassment.
Avoidance- Avoidance is very commonly observed with malodor person. Affected persons are intentionally avoided by their classmates, roommate and office colleagues, friends, family etc.
Self-esteem- People sometime get highly depressed

that they lost their self-confidence and self belief. Sometime they cannot self-estimate their own breath status. Very low self esteem is usually accompanied with this situation.

Anxiety- Depression generates frustration on the affected subject's mind and thus frustration gets evolved into severe anxiety. Anxiety to the social awareness and social reaction of the people is usually associated with affected subjects.

Outburst- Sometimes the subject may lose control on their mind and it comes out by an outburst on his/ her close relative. This usually happens due to chronic frustration and insecurity.

Obsessive compulsive disorder- Due to fear of ignorance, avoidance and rejection severely affected person may develop some recitative takes like excessive cleaning of mouth etc. converting theses habits into obsessive compulsive disorder further which could be a difficult psychological problem to cure.

Oral malodor or fetor exore is a foul or offensive odor emanating from the mouth and is a frequent cause for patients to seek treatment.

Intraoral and extraoral factors have been attributed to halitosis. In most cases bad breath originates from the oral cavity itself. Poor oral hygiene, periodontal pockets, faulty restorations, dry sockets, unclean dentures and abscesses are often overlooked as potential sources of Volatile Sulfur Compounds. Volatile Sulfur Compounds result from proteolytic degradation by anaerobic oral microorganisms found abundantly in periodontal pockets and on the surface of the tongue. A variety of methods like organoleptic assessment, gas chromatography, and sulfide monitoring have been used to assess oral malodor.

To date, no specific treatment modality has shown consistent results in all cases because of the varied causes for oral malodor. Research is still underway to find a cure for this socially embarrassing problem. In most cases, good professional oral care combined with a daily regimen of oral hygiene, including interdental cleaning, tongue cleaning, and the optional use of a mouthrinse, can lead to improvement. Patient education about oral hygiene practices is crucial for treatment to be effective. With increasing demand for dental care, and with continuing advances in dental education and research, there may be a greater potential for the dentists to play a prominent role in the prevention and control of oral malodor.

1. **Rayman** S, Almas K. Halitosis among Racially Diverse Populations: an Update. Int *J Dent Hyg.2008;6(1):2-7.*

2. **Winkel EG**. Halitosis Control. In: Lindhe J, Lang NP, Karring T, editors. *Clinical Peridontology and Implant Dentistry. 5th ed. Iowa: Blackwell Publishing; 2008. p. 1325-40.*

3. **Van den Broek AM, Feenstra L, de BaatC.** A Review of the Current Literature on Aetiology and Measurement Methods of Halitosis. *J Dent.2007;35(8):627-35.*

4. **Brening RH, Sulser GF, Fosdick LS**. The Determination of Halitosis by Use of the Osmoscope and the Cryoscopic Method. *J Dent Res 1939;18:127-132.*

5. **Gnanasekhar JD.** Aetiology, Diagnosis and Management of Halitosis- a Review. *Perio 2007;4(3):203–214.*

6. **Pratibha PK, Bhat KM, Bhat GS.** Oral malodor: a Review of the Literature. *J Dent Hyg. 2006;80(3):1-9.*

7. **Newman MG, Takei HH, Klokkevold PR, Carranza FA**, editors. *Carranza's Clinical Periodontology. 10^{th}ed. St. Louis: Saunders Company; 2009. p. 330-42.*

8. **Murata T, Rahardjo A, Fujiyama Y, Yamaga T, Hanada M, Yaegaki K, et al.** Development of

a Compact and Simple Gas Chromatography for Oral Malodor Measurement. *J Periodontol. 2006;77(7):1142-7.*

9. **Krespi YP, Slatkine M, Marchenko M, Protic J.** Lethal Photosensitization of Oral Pathogens Via Red-Filtered Halogen Lamp. *Oral Dis.2005;11(1):92-5.*

10. **ADA Council on Scientific Affairs**. Oral Malodor. *J Am Dent Assoc.2003;134(2):209-14.*

11. **Hughes FJ, McNab R.** Oral Malodour-A Review. *Arch Oral Biol.2008;53 (1):S1-7.*

12. **Rosenberg M, Septon I, Eli I, Bar-Ness R, Gelernter I, Brenner S, et al.** Halitosis Measurement by an Industrial Sulphide Monitor. *J Periodontol.1991;62(8):487-9.*

13. **Bornstein MM, Kislig K, Hoti BB, Seemann R, Lussi A**. Prevalence of Halitosis in the Population of the City of Bern, Switzerland: A Study Comparing Self-Reported and Clinical Data. *Eur J Oral Sci.2009;117(3):261-7.*

14. **Honda E**. Oral Microbial Flora and Oral Malodor of the Institutionalised Elderly in Japan. *Gerodontology. 2001;18(2):65-72.*

15. **Seemann R, Bizhang M, Djamchidi C, Kage A, Nachnani S.** The Proportion of Pseudo-Halitosis patients in a Multidisciplinary Breath Malodour Consultation. *Int Dent J. 2006;56(2):77-81.*

16. **Nadanovsky P, Carvalho LB, PoncedeLeon A.**

Oral Malodor and Its Association with Age and Sex in a General Population in Brazil. *OralDis.2007;13(1):105-9.*

17. **Bornstein MM, Stocker BL, Seemann R, Bürgin WB, Lussi A.** Prevalence of Halitosis in Young Male Adults: A Study In Swiss Army Recruits Comparing Self-Reported and Clinical Data.*J Periodontol. 2009;80(1):24-31.*

18. **Quirynen M, Dadamio J, VandenVelde S, DeSmit M, Dekeyser C, Van Tornout M, et al.** Characteristics of 2000 patients Who Visited a Halitosis Clinic. *J Clin Periodontol. 2009;36(11):970-5.*

19. **Kleinberg I, Westbay G**. Oral Malodor. *Crit Rev Oral Biol Med.1990;1;247-259.*

20. **Tangerman A, Winkel EG.** Intra and Extra-Oral Halitosis: Finding of a New Form of Extra-oral Blood-Borne Halitosis Caused by Dimethyl Sulphide. *J Clin Periodontol. 2007;34(9):748-55.*

21. **Faveri M, Feres M, Shibli JA, Hayacibara RF, Hayacibara MM, de Figueiredo LC.** Microbiota of the Dorsum of the Tongue after Plaque Accumulation: an Experimental Study in Humans. *J Periodontol.2006;77(9):1539-46.*

22. **McNamara TF, Alexander JF, Lee M.** The Role of Microorganisms in the Production of Oral Malodor. *Oral Surg Oral Med Oral Pathol. 1972;34(1):41-8.*

23. **Scully C, Greenman J.** Halitosis (Breath Odor). *Periodontol 2000.2008;48:66-75.*

24. **Kleinberg I, Codipilly M.** Modeling of the Oral Malodor System and Methods of Analysis. *Quintessence Int. 1999;30(5):357-69.*

25. **Tonzetich J, Richter VJ.** Evaluation of Volatile Odoriferous Components of Saliva. *Arch Oral Biol. 1964;9:39-46.*

26. **Goldberg S, Kozlovsky A, Gordon D, Gelernter I, Sintov A, Rosenberg M.** Cadaverine as a Putative Component of Oral Malodor. *J Dent Res.1994;73(6):1168-72.*

27. **Tonzetich J.** Production and Origin of Oral Malodor: A Review of Mechanisms and Methods of Analysis. *J Periodontol. 1977;48(1):13-20.*

28. **Scully C, el-Maaytah M, Porter SR, Greenman J.** Breathodor: Etiopathogenesis, Assessment and Management. *Eur J Oral Sci.1997;105(4):287-93.*

29. **Ratcliff PA, Johnson PW**. The Relationship Between Oral Malodor, Gingivitis, and Periodontitis. A review. *J Periodontol. 1999;70(5):485-9.*

30. **Loesche WJ, Kazor C.** Microbiology and Treatment of Halitosis. *Periodontol2000. 2002;28:256-79.*

31. **Wu AP.** Halitosis. *Oral Surg. 1982;54(2):221-3.*

32. **Gupta PV.** Differential Diagnosis of Dental

Diseases.1ˢᵗ ed. Delhi: Jaypee Brothers Medical Publishers (P) Ltd.;2008. *p.201-15.*

33. **Bogdasarian RS.** Halitosis. *Otolaryngol Clin North Am. 1986;19(1):111-7.*

34. **Yaegaki K, Coil JM.** Examination, Classification, and Treatment of Halitosis; Clinical Perspectives. *J Can Dent Assoc. 2000;66(5):257-61.*

35. **Lee SS, Zhang WU, Li Y.** Halitosis Update- A Review of Causes, Diagnoses, and Treatments. *J Can Dent Assoc. 2007 Jul;35(4):259-68.*

36. **Holmstrup P, Westergaard J.** Necrotizing periodontal disease *Clinical Peridontology and Implant Dentistry. 5ᵗʰ ed. Iowa: Blackwell Publishing; 2008. p.459-474.*

37. **Marucha PT.** Acute Gingival Infections. *Carranza's Clinical Periodontology.10ᵗʰed. St. Louis: Saunders Company; 2009. p. 391-403.*

38. **Navazesh M, Kumar SK.** Xerostomia: Prevalence, Diagnosis, and Management. *Compend Contin Educ Dent. 2009;30(6):326-8, 331-2.*

39. **Haraszthy VI, Zambon JJ, Sreenivasan PK, Zambon MM, Gerber D, Rego R, et al.** Identification of Oral Bacterial Species Associated with Halitosis. *J Am Dent Assoc. 2007;138(8):1113-20.*

40. **Cortelli JR, Barbosa MD, Westphal MA.**

Halitosis: A Review of Associated Factors and Therapeutic Approach. *Braz Oral Res. 2008;22(Suppl 1):44-54.*

41. **Amler M.** Disturbed Healing of Extraction Wounds. *J Oral Implantol.1999;25(3):179-84.*

42. **Lu DP.** Halitosis: An Etiologic Classification, A Treatment Approach, and Prevention. *Oral Surg Oral Med Oral Pathol. 1982;54(5):521-6.*

43. **Rio AC, Franchi-Teixeira AR, Nicola EM.** Relationship Between the Presence of Tonsilloliths and Halitosis in Patients with Chronic Caseous Tonsillitis. *Br Dent J. 2008 Jan 26;204(2):E4.*

44. **Suzuki N, Yoneda M, Naito T, Iwamoto T, Masuo Y, Yamada K, et al.** Detection of Helicobacter pylori DNA in the Saliva of Patients Complaining of Halitosis. *J Med Microbiol. 2008;57(12):1553-9.*

45. **Mitchell SC.** Trimethylaminuria(Fish-OdourSyndrome) and Oral Malodour. *Oral Dis. 2005;11(1):10-3.*

46. **Preti G, Clark L, Cowart BJ, Feldman RS, Lowry LD, Weber E, et al.** Non-Oral Etiologies of Oral Malodor and Altered Chemosensation. *J Periodontol. 1992;63(9):790-6.*

47. **De Boever EH, Loesche WJ.** Assessing the Contribution of Anaerobic Microflora of the Tongue to Oral Malodor. *J Am Dent Assoc.1995;126(10):1384-93.*

48. **Calil CM, Lima PO, Bernardes CF, Groppo FC, Bado F, Marcondes FK.** Influence of Gender and Menstrual Cycle on Volatile Sulphur Compounds Production. *Arch Oral Biol. 2008;53(12):1107-12.*

49. **Calil CM, Marcondes FK**. Influence of Anxiety on the Production of Oral Volatile Sulfur Compounds. *Life Sci. 2006 Jul 10;79(7):660-4.*

50. **Morita M, Wang HL.** Relationship between Sulcular Sulfide Level and Oral Malodor in Subjects with Periodontal Disease. *J Periodontol.2001;72(1):79-84.*

51. **Figueiredo LC, Rosetti EP, Marcantonio E, Marcantonio RA, Salvador SL**. The Relationship of Oral Malodor in Patients With or Without Periodontal Disease. *J Periodontol. 2002;73(11):1338-42.*

52. **Lee CH, Kho HS, Chung SC, Lee SW, Kim YK**. The Relationship Between Volatile Sulfur Compounds and Major Halitosis-Inducing Factors. *J Periodontol. 2003;74(1):32-7.*

53. **Tsai CC, Chou HH, Wu TL, Yang YH, Ho KY, Wu YM, et al.** The Levels of Volatile Sulfur Compounds in Mouth Air From Patients With Chronic Periodontitis. *J Periodontal Res. 2008;43(2):186-93.*

54. **Calil C, Liberato FL, Pereira AC, deCastroMeneghim M, Goodson JM, Groppo FC et al.** The Relationship between Volatile

Sulphur Compounds, Tongue Coating and Periodontal Disease. *Int J Dent Hyg.* *2009;7(4):251-5.*

55. **Rizzo AA.** Histologic and Immunologic Evaluation of Antigen Penetration into Oral Tissues after Topical Application. *J Periodontol. 1970;41(4):210-3.*

56. **Ng W, Tonzetich J.** Effect of Hydrogen Sulphide and Methyl Mercaptan on the Permeability of Oral Mucosa. *J Dent Res 1984;63:994-997.*

57. **Imai T, Ii H, Yaegaki K, Murata T, Sato T, Kamoda T.** Oral Malodorous Compound Inhibits Osteoblast Proliferation. *J Periodontol2009;80(12):2028-34.*

58. **Miyazaki H, Sakao S, Katoh Y, Takehara T.** Correlation between Volatile Sulphur Compounds and Certain Oral Health Measurements in the General Population. *J Periodontol. 1995;66(8):679-84.*

59. **MantillaGómez S, Danser MM, Sipos PM, Rowshani B, vanderVelden U, vanderWeijden GA.** Tongue Coating and Salivary Bacterial Counts in Healthy/Gingivitis Subjects and Periodontitis Patients. *J Clin Periodontol.2001;28(10):970-8.* **Winkel EG.** Clinical effects of a new mouthrinse containing chlorhexidine. *J Clin Periodontol. 2003;30(3):201-3.*

60. **Oho T, Yoshida Y, Shimazaki Y, Yamashita Y, Koga T.** Characteristics of Patients Complaining of Halitosis and the Usefulness of Gas Chromatography for Diagnosing Halitosis. *Oral Surg Oral Med Oral Pathol Oral Radiol Endod. 2001;91(5):531-4*

61. **Nachnani S, Majerus G, Lenton P, Hodges J, Magallanes E.** Effects of Training on Odor Judges Scoring Intensity.*Oral Dis. 2005;11 (Suppl 1):40-4.*

62. **Kim DJ, Lee JY, Kho HS, Chung JW, Park HK, Kim YK.** A New Organoleptic Testing Method for Evaluating halitosis. *J Periodontol.2009;80(1):93-7.*

63. **Halimeter:** used in the diagnosis and treatment of chronic halitosis. Available from:*http://www.halimeter.com/.* [last accessed on 27.05.2017]

64. **Oral Chroma:** A Halitosis Measuring Device [Internet]. Osaka(JP): Abimedical Corp.; c2008. Available from: *http://www.abilit-medical-and-environmental.jp/en/medical/index.html* [last accessed on 12.06.2017]

65. **Ueno M, Shinada K, Yanagisawa T, Mori C, Yokoyama S, Furukawa S, et al.** Clinical Oral Malodor Measurement with a Portable Sulfide Monitor. *Oral Dis. 2008 Apr;14(3):264-9.*

66. **Sanz M, Newman MG, Quirymen M.** Advanced Diagnostics Aids. In: Newman MG, Takei HH, Klokkevold PR, Carranza FA, editors. *Carranza's Clinical Periodontology. 10th ed. St. Louis: Saunders Company;2009.p.579-601.*

67. **Tanaka M, Anguri H, Nonaka A, Kataoka K, Nagata H, Kita J et al.** Clinical Assessment of Oral Malodor by the Electronic Nose System. *J Dent Res. 2004;83(4):317-21.*

68. **Quirynen M, Zhao H, Avontroodt P, Soers C, Pauwels M, Coucke W, et al.** A Salivary Incubation Test for Evaluation of Oral Malodor: A Pilot Study. *J Periodontol. 2003;74(7):937-44.*

69. **Morita M, Musinski DL, Wang HL.** Assessment of Newly Developed Tongue Sulfide Probe for Detecting Oral Malodor. *J Clin Periodontol.2001;28(5):494-6.*

70. **Shimura M, Yasuno Y, Iwakura M, Shimada Y, Sakai S, Suzuki K, et al.** A New Monitor with a Zinc-Oxide Thin Film Semi conductor Sensor for the Measurement of Volatile Sulfur Compounds in Mouth Air. *J Periodontol.1996;67(4):396-402.*

71. **Rosenberg M, Barki M, Goldberg S.** The Antimicrobial Effect of Mouthrinsing as Measured Using the "Oratest". *J Dent Res.1996;68(4):655-662).*

72. **Rosenberg M, Kozlovsky A, Gelernter I, Cherniak O, Gabbay J, Baht R et al. Self-Estimation of Oral Malodor.** *J Dent Res. 1995;74(9):1577-82.*

73. **Rosenberg M, Kulkarni GV, Bosy A, McCulloch CA.** Reproducibility and Sensitivity of Oral Malodor Measurements with a Portable Sulphide Monitor. *J Dent Res. 1991;70(11):1436-40.*

74. **Kozlovsky A, Gordon D, Gelernter I, Loesche WJ, Rosenberg M.** Correlation Between the BANA test and Oral Malodor Parameters. *J Dent Res. 1994;73(5):1036-42.*

75. **Rosenberg M, Kozlovsky A, Wind Y, Mindel E**. Self-Assessment of Oral Malodor 1 Year Following Initial Consultation. *Quintessence Int.1999;30(5):324-7.*

76. **Furne J, Majerus G, Lenton P, Springfield J, Levitt DG, Levitt MD**. Comparison of Volatile Sulfur Compound Concentrations Measured with a Sulfide Detector vs. Gas Chromatography. *J Dent Res. 2002;81(2):140-3.*

77. **Tanaka M, Anguri H, Nishida N, Ojima M, Nagata H, Shizukuishi S.** Reliability of Clinical Parameters for Predicting the Outcome of Oral Malodor Treatment. *J Dent Res. 2003;82(7):518-22.*

78. **Kato H, Yoshida A, Awano S, Ansai T, Takehara T.** Quantitative Detection of Volatile

Sulfur Compound-Producing Microorganisms in Oral Specimens using Real-Time PCR. *Oral Dis. 2005;11(1):67-71.*

79. **Phillips M, Cataneo RN, Greenberg J, Munawar M, Nachnani S, Samtani S.** Pilot study of a Breath Test for Volatile Organic Compounds Associated with Oral Malodor: Evidence for the Role of Oxidative Stress. *Oral Dis.2005;11(1):32-4.*

80. **Iwanicka-Grzegorek K, Lipkowska E, Kepa J, Michalik J, Wierzbicka M.** Comparison of Ninhydrin Method of Detecting Amine Compounds with Other Methods of Halitosis Detection. *Oral Dis. 2005;11(Suppl 1):37-9.*

81. **Hunter CM, Niles HP, Vazquez J, Kloos C, Subramanyam R, Williams MI, et al.** Breath Odor Evaluation by Detection of Volatile Sulfur Compounds-Correlation with Organoleptic Odor Ratings. *Oral Dis.2005;11(1):48-50.*

82. **Roldán S, Herrera D, O'Connor A, González I, Sanz M.** A Combined Therapeutic Approach to Manage Oral Halitosis: a 3-Month Prospective Case Series. *J Periodontol. 2005 Jun;76(6):1025-33.*

83. **Seemann R, Kison A, Bizhang M, Zimmer S.** Effectiveness of Mechanical Tongue Cleaning on Oral Levels of Volatile Sulfur Compounds. *J Am Dent Assoc. 2001;132(9):1263-7.*

84. **Winkel EG, Roldán S, VanWinkelhoff AJ,**

Herrera D, Sanz M. Clinical Effects of a New Mouthrinse Containing Chlorhexidine, Cetylpyridinium Chloride and Zinc-Lactate on Oral Halitosis. A Dual-Center, Double-Blind Placebo-Controlled Study. *J Clin Periodontol. 2003;30(4):300-6.*

85. **Bordas A, McNab R, Staples AM, Bowman J, Kanapka J, Bosma MP**. Impact of Different Tongue Cleaning Methods on the Bacterial Load of the Tongue Dorsum.*Arch Oral Biol. 2008;53(1):S13-8*

86. **Outhouse TL, Al-Alawi R, Fedorowicz Z, Keenan JV.** Tongue Scraping for Treating Halitosis. *Cochrane Database Syst Rev. 2006;19(2):CD005519.*

87. **Quirynen M, Zhao H, Soers C, Dekeyser C, Pauwels M, Coucke W, et al.** The Impact of Periodontal Therapy and the Adjunctive Effect of Antiseptics on Breath Odor-related Outcome Variables: a Double-Blind Randomized Study. *J Periodontol. 2005;76(5):705-12.*

88. **VanSteenberghe D, Avontroodt P, Peeters W, Pauwels M, CouckeW, LijnenA, et al**. Effect of Different Mouthrinses on Morning Breath. *J Periodontol. 2001;72(9):1183-91.*

89. **Carvalho MD, Tabchoury CM, Cury JA, Toledo S, Nogueira-Filho GR.** Impact of Mouthrinses on Morning Bad Breath in Healthy

Subjects. *J Clin Periodontol. 2004;31(2):85-90.*

90. **Bosy A, Kulkarni GV, Rosenberg M, McCulloch CA.** Relationship of Oral Malodor to Periodontitis: Evidence of Independence in Discrete Subpopulations. *J Periodontol. 1994;65(1):37-46.*

91. **Pitts G, Brogdon C, Hu L, Masurat T, Pianotti R, Schumann P.**Mechanism of Action of an Antiseptic, Anti-Odor Mouthwash. *J Dent Res.1983;62(6):738-42.*

92. **Young A, Jonski G, Rölla G.** A Study of Triclosan and its Solubilizers as Inhibitors of Oral Malodour. *J Clin Periodontol. 2002;29(12):1078-81.*

93. **Moran J, Addy M.** The Effects of a Cetyl pyridinium Chloride Prebrushing Rinse as an Adjunct to Oral Hygiene and Gingival Health. *J Periodontol.1991;62(9):562-4.*

94. **Young A, Jonski G, Rölla G.** Inhibition of Orally Produced Volatile Sulfur Compounds by Zinc, Chlorhexidine or Cetyl pyridinium Chloride— Effect of Concentration. *Eur J Oral Sci. 2003t;111(5):400-4.*

95. **Frascella J, Gilbert R, Fernandez P.** Odor Reduction Potential of a Chlorine Dioxide Mouthrinse. *J Clin Dent. 1998;9(2):39-42.*

96. **Richter JL.** Diagnosis and Treatment of Halitosis.*Compend Contin Educ Dent. 1996 Apr;17(4):370-2*

97. **Roldán S, Winkel EG, Herrera D, Sanz M, Van Winkelhoff AJ**. The Effects of a New Mouthrinse Containing Chlorhexidine, Cetylpyridinium Chloride and Zinc Lactate on the Microflora of Oral Halitosis Patients: A Dual-Centre, Double-Blind Placebo-Controlled Study. *J Clin Periodontol.2003 May;30(5):427-34.*

98. **Roldán S, Herrera D, Santa-Cruz I, O'Connor A, González I, Sanz M.** Comparative effects of different chlorhexidine mouth-rinse formulations on volatile sulphur compounds and salivary bacterial counts. *J Clin Periodontol.2004 Dec;31(12):1128-34.*

99. **Burton JP, Chilcott CN, Tagg JR.** The Rationale and Potential for the Reduction of Oral Malodour using Streptococcus Salivarius Probiotics. *Oral Dis. 2005;11(1):29-31.*

100. **Wåler SM**. The Effect of Zinc-Containing Chewing Gum on Volatile Sulfur-Containing Compounds in the Oral Cavity. *Acta Odontol Scand.1997;55(3):198-200.*

101. **Reingewirtz Y, Girault O, Reingewirtz N, Senger B, Tenenbaum H**. Mechanical Effects and Volatile Sulfur Compound-Reducing Effects of Chewing gums: Comparison Between Test and Base Gums and a Control Group. *Quintessence Int. 1999;30(5):319-23.*

102.   **Rösing CK, Jonski G, Rølla G**. Comparative Analysis of Some Mouthrinses on the Production of Volatile Sulfur-Containing Compounds. *Acta Odontol Scand. 2002;60(1):10-2.*

103.   **Niles HP, Hunter C, Vazquez J, Williams MI, Cummins D.** The Clinical Comparison of Triclosan/Copolymer/fluoride Dentifrice vs a Breath- Freshening Dentifrice in Reducing Breath Odor Overnight: a Crossover Study. *Oral Dis. 2005;11(1):54-6.*

104.   **Vazquez J, Pilch S, Williams MI, Cummins D.** Clinical Efficacy of a Triclosan/Copolymer/NaF Dentifrice and a Commercially Available Breath-Freshening Dentifrice on Hydrogen Sulfide-Forming Bacteria. *Oral Dis.2005;11(Suppl 1):64-6.*

105.   **Hu D, Zhang YP, Petrone M, Volpe AR, Devizio W, Giniger M.** Clinical Effectiveness of a Triclosan/copolymer/sodium Fluoride Dentifrice in Controlling Oral Malodor:a 3-Week Clinical Trial. *Oral Dis.2005;11(1):51-3.*

106.   **Haas AN, Silveira EM, Rösing CK.** Effect of Tongue Cleansing on Morning Oral Malodor in Periodontally Healthy Individuals. *Oral Health Prev Dent.2007;5(2):89-94.*

107.   **Calil C , Liberto FL, Grappo FC.** The relationship between volatile sulphur compounds, tongue coating and periodontal disease. Int J Dent

Hygiene 2009;7:251-255

108.   **Saad S, Greenman J, Shawz H**. Comparative effects of various commercially available mouthrinse formulations on oral malodour .Oral Diseases 2011;17:180–186

109.   **Raangs GC , Winkel EG , van Winkelhoff AJ.** In vitro antimicrobial effects of two antihalitosis mouth rinses on oral pathogens and human tongue microbiota. Int J Dent Hygiene 2013;11:203–207.

110.   **F. Yang, S. Huang, T. He, C. Catrenich, F. Teng, C. Bo, J. Chen, J. Liu, J. Li, Y. Song, R. Li, and J. Xu** Microbial Basis of Oral Malodor Development in Humans. *J Dent Res 2013;* 92(12):1106-1112

111.   **Jeronimo M. Oliveira-Neto, Sandra Sato, Vinícius Pedrazzi.** How to deal with morning bad breath: A randomized, crossover clinical trial. J Periodon 2013;17(6):45-46

112.   **Seida Erovic Ademovski, Peter Lingström, Edwin Winkel, Albert Tangerman G, Persson R, Renvert S**. Comparison of different treatment modalities for oral halitosis. Acta Odontologica Scandinavica 2012; 70: 224–233